Keto For Women Over 50

Your Tailor-Made Program to Deflate the Belly, Abdominal Fat, and Tone the Muscles. Lose Weight Easily with the Keto Diet to Experience a Happy Menopause

Keli Bay

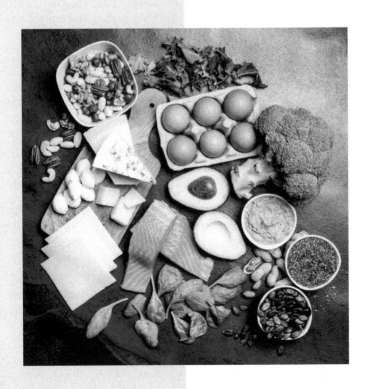

Table of Contents

Introduction

You Can Have A Perfect Body Even At 50

It's not in your brain, women - people don't live in an equivalent world with regards to muscle to fat ratio. Men, with their taller bodies and profound muscle tissues and bones, lay pronounce to snappier digestion. At adolescence, young ladies put on fat, and young men apply on muscle. From breastfeeding to preparation, young ladies have and need more noteworthy fats than men. In this part, we will investigate the advantages and inconveniences of IF and how ladies more than 50 should move toward the eating regimen.

At the point when you quick, your body consumes fat rather than sugar for vitality, which brings about fat misfortune and gives your mind a lift.

Like a car, your body needs fuel to run; Food is that fuel. During digestion, the stomach breaks down the carbohydrates in the sugar that the cells use for energy, to "feed," so to speak. If your cells do not use all the available glucose, eventually, the fat is retained, as you have already guessed. During fasting, your cells go from using glucose as the main source of fuel to consuming fat.

Therefore, fat deposits, mainly triglycerides, are burned for energy. Therefore, research has found that IF can help you lose weight while maintaining muscle mass.

It gives protection from epileptic seizures, Alzheimer's sickness and other neurodegenerative issues.

Exactly when your body uses fat stores for imperativeness, it releases unsaturated fats called ketones into the circulatory framework. Ketones assume a job in weight reduction yet have been appeared to keep up cerebrum work, giving even some protection from epileptic seizures, Alzheimer's malady and other neurodegenerative issues.

For example, a study in older adults with mild cognitive impairment found that an increase in ketones improved memory in just six weeks. Such benefits can occur because ketones secrete brain-derived neurotrophic factor (BDNF), which improves neuronal connections, especially in areas involved in memory and learning.

Studies have shown that if it stimulates the growth of new neurons in the brain.

When you fast, your insulin levels drop, while your human growth hormone and norepinephrine levels rise, which helps you weaken and withstand chronic diseases.

Put simply, we get a torrent of insulin when we eat, while levels drop when we fast. Insulin regulates whether additional glucose from digestion is stored in the body in the form of fat, another reason why IF can contribute to weight loss.

Research shows that IF dramatically lowers insulin and can reduce hyperinsulinemia, as well as improve insulin sensitivity. In animal studies, IF was tested for both diabetes prevention and reversal.

Research also suggests that when insulin is low, and the body registers an increase in transcription factors, which control metabolism-related genes. Finally, this process can change the expression of genes in favor of healthy aging and longevity.

IF also appears to decrease insulin-like growth factors, a genetic marker for diseases such as cancer.

Studies show the arrival of HGH. This is noteworthy on the grounds that, as we become more seasoned, our bodies respond and may bring down the creation of HGH, and this is related to expanded fat tissue and loss of bulk. Exploration of the impact of HGH on body structure proposes that it can assist subjects with getting more fit without losing muscle.

This peak of this neurotransmitter, which you can call it also the stress hormone, contributes to the positive impact of IF on metabolism and helps the body break down fat as a fuel.

Intermittent fasting in what society calls it, interchange day fasting, despite the fact that there is absolutely a few minor departures from this eating regimen. The Journal of Clinical Nutrition executed a glance at nowadays that enlisted 16 hefty guys and females on a 10-week program. On the fasting days, members benefited from food to 25% of their assessed power needs. The remainder of the time, they got healthful directing; notwithstanding, were not, at this point given a particular core value to follow all through this time.

As expected, the participants misplaced weight because of this observe, however, what researchers determined thrilling have been some unique changes. The topics had been all still obese after simply ten weeks, but they'd shown development in cholesterol, LDL-systolic blood pressure, triglycerides, and cholesterol. What made this a thrilling find turned into that most people must lose greater weight than these take a look at participants before seeing the equal changes. It was a captivating find which has spurred an exceptional range of human beings to try fasting.

Intermittent fasting for girls has some useful effects. What makes it especially essential for older girls who are trying to lose weight is that they have a far higher fats proportion in our bodies. When trying to lose weight, the frame, on the whole, burns through carbohydrate stores with the first 6 hours and then begins to burn fats. Women over 50 who are following a healthy food plan and exercise plan may be struggling with stubborn fats, but fasting is a realistic technique to this.

Chapter 1
The Ketogenic Diet: Why It Is Called Ketogenic

People who engage in Keto diet, particularly those aged 50 and older, are said to reap various potential health benefits including:

Improved Physical And Mental Strength

At the point when a person establishes more developed, vitality levels that fall for an assortment of ecological and organic reasons. Disciples to the Keto diet regularly experience a lift in quality and imperativeness. One explanation the event is on the grounds that the body consumes abundance fat, which is combined into vitality thusly.

Metabolism

Maturing individuals regularly experience a more slow digestion than they have encountered in their more youthful days. Long haul keto health food nuts experience expanded blood glucose control, which may improve their metabolic rates.

Protection Against Specific Diseases

Keto dieters over 50 years of age may reduce their risk of developing diseases such as diabetes, mental disorders such as Alzheimer's, various cardiovascular diseases, various types of cancer, Parkinson's disease, non-alcoholic fatty liver disease (NAFLD) and multiple sclerosis.

Good news from the technical description of the ketosis cycle mentioned earlier, reveals the increased energy of the youth as a consequence and because of the use of fat as a source of fuel, the body can go through a phase where signals can be misinterpreted so that the mTOR signal is blocked and a loss of insulin is apparent where aging is stated to be slowed down.

Multiple studies have commonly recognized for years that what cab help you slow your aging process is through caloric restriction and even increasing the lifespan. With the ketogenic diet, it is important to influence anti-aging without increasing calories. The periodic form of fasting used with the keto diet may also impact vascular aging.

The Ketogenic Diet

The Ketogenic Diet follows a simple principle: keep your food consumption low-carb and high-fat. So basically, being on the diet means eating fewer carbohydrates and adding more fats in your daily meals. Do not be confused. When we say "fat" we are not talking about the literal kind that is attached to your body. Fat has gotten a bad reputation nowadays, but "fat" the nutrient is actually very different from the "fat" that makes your clothes fit tight.

Good fats are the kind you get from avocado, nuts, and fish. For example, there are the omega-3 and omega-6 fatty acids that help you lose weight, get better heart health, and have excellent hair and nails.

Naturally, the question that is asked about the Keto Diet is why so many of your friends who are on the Keto Diet seem to be losing so much weight so quickly. The reality is that in the first three to six months on the Keto diet, the body is dropping a tremendous amount of weight because of how the diet is forcing the body to draw energy. Remember how it was said earlier how the body likes to use blood sugar because blood sugar is an easy way to draw energy without using too much energy? Well, what happens when the blood sugar is not in large supply?

This is the essence of weight loss with the Keto Diet. The reality is that weight loss occurs because it takes a lot of calories to burn a single fat cell compared to the calories needed to use blood sugar. The same is true for the protein that is in the body. There is also a psychological element at play here. Carbs can be empty calories and they are really easy to convert into energy – in fact, as you are chewing a piece of bread the body is getting the nutrients from it, whereas if you are eating something that is denser – like meat – then what happens is the digestion occurs in the stomach. It takes much energy to digest a high fat, high protein diet. And – here is the good news – who does not like to have a diet where they can eat things that they love?! This is the great part about the Keto Diet. The high fat and high protein that goes into the diet provides what the body needs in calories to fire up the burning of the fat cells that are critical to losing weight.

When a human fast intermittently or is developed on a keto diet, it is suspected that BHB or Beta-Hydroxybutyrate causes anti-aging results.

Very little in carbs and regularly solid in fats or potentially proteins, ketogenic eats less are utilized effectively for weight reduction during overweight and coronary illness care. Be that as it may, a significant note in the article was that "Results on the effect of such weight control plans on cardiovascular hazard factors are questionable" and "furthermore, these eating regimens are not totally protected and might be related to some unfriendly occasions. More is required than simply investigating this eating routine, points of interest, constructive outcomes, and reactions, especially in matured grown-ups on the Internet. One ought to address their clinical expert about explicit concerns.

Even before we talk about how to do keto – it is important to first consider why this diet works. What happens to your body to make you lose weight?

As you probably know, the body uses food as an energy source. Everything you eat is turned into energy, so that you can get up and do whatever you need to accomplish for the day. The main energy source is sugar so what happens is that you eat something, the body breaks it down into sugar, and the sugar is processed into energy. Typically, the "sugar" is taken directly from the food you eat so if you eat just the right amount of food, then your body is fueled for the whole day. If you eat too much, then the sugar is stored in your body – hence the accumulation of fat.

But what happens if you eat less food? This is where the Ketogenic Diet comes in. You see, the process of creating sugar from food is usually faster if the food happens to be rich in carbohydrates. Bread, rice, grain, pasta – all of these are carbohydrates and they are the easiest food types to turn into energy.

So, the Ketogenic Diet is all about reducing the number of carbohydrates you eat. Does this mean you will not get the kind of energy you need for the day? Of course not! It only means that now, your body must find other possible sources of energy. Do you know where they will be getting that energy? Your stored body fat!

So, here is the situation – you are eating fewer carbohydrates every day. To keep you energetic, the body breaks down the stored fat and turns them into molecules called ketone bodies. The process of turning the fat into ketone bodies is called "Ketosis" and obviously – this is where the name of the Ketogenic Diet comes from. The ketone bodies take the place of glucose in keeping you energetic. If you keep your carbohydrates reduced, the body will keep getting its energy from your body fat.

Sounds Simple, Right?

The Ketogenic Diet is often praised for its simplicity and when you look at it properly, the process is straightforward. The Science behind the effectivity of the diet is also well-documented and has been proven multiple times by different medical fields. For example, an article on Diet Assessment by Harvard provided a lengthy discussion on how the Ketogenic Diet works and why it is so effective for those who choose to use this diet.

But Fat Is the Enemy...Or Is It?

No – fat is NOT the enemy. Unfortunately, years of bad science told us that fat is something you must avoid – but it is actually an extremely helpful thing for weight loss! Even before we move forward with this guide, we will have to discuss exactly what "healthy fats" are, and why they are the good guys. To do this, we need to make a distinction between the different kinds of fat. You have probably heard of them before and it is a little bit confusing at first. We will try to go through them as simply as possible:

Saturated fat. This is the kind you want to avoid. They are also called "solid fat" because each molecule is packed with hydrogen atoms. Simply put, it is the kind of fat that can easily cause a blockage in your body. It can raise cholesterol levels and lead to heart problems or a stroke. Saturated fat is something you can find in meat, dairy products, and other processed food items. Now, you are probably wondering: isn't the Ketogenic Diet packed with saturated fat? The answer is: not necessarily. You will find in the recipes given that the Ketogenic Diet promotes primarily unsaturated fat or healthy fat. While there are many meat recipes on the list, most of these recipes contain healthy fat sources.

Unsaturated Fat. These are the ones dubbed as a healthy fat. They are the kind of fat you find in avocado, nuts, and other ingredients you usually find in Keto-friendly recipes. They are known to lower blood cholesterol and come in two types: polyunsaturated and monounsaturated. Both are good for your body, but the benefits slightly vary, depending on what you are consuming.

Polyunsaturated fat. These are perhaps the best on the list. You know about omega-3 fatty acids, right? They are often suggested for people who have heart problems and are recognized as the "healthy" kind of fat. Well, they fall under the category of polyunsaturated fat and are known for reducing risks of heart disease by as much as 19 percent. This is according to a study titled: Effects on coronary heart diseases of increased poly-unsaturated fat in lieu of saturated fat: systematic assessment & meta-analysis of randomized controlled tests. So where do you get these polyunsaturated fats? You can get them mostly from vegetable and seed oils. These are ingredients you can almost always find in Ketogenic Recipes such as olive oil, coconut oil, and more. If you need more convincing, you should also know that omega-3 fatty acids are a kind of polyunsaturated fats and you will find them in deep sea fish like tuna, herring, and salmon.

Carbohydrates in a regular meal generally make up most

of the calories. Also, as it is easier to absorb, the body is inclined to use the carbohydrate as energy. Therefore, the diet's proteins and fats are more likely to be stored.

The body resorts to its stored fat content because of this apparent shortage. It makes a shift from a consumer of carbohydrates to a fat burner. However, in the recently ingested meal, the body does not use the fats, but instead stores them for another round of ketosis.

The body still needs a constant supply of energy during fasting periods-such as during ketosis, between meals and during sleep. You have these times in your normal day, so you need to consume enough fat to use your body as energy. A keto diet's main goal is to mimic the body's hunger state. By restricting and severely reducing the intake of carbohydrates, keto diets deprive the body of its preferred immediate and easily convertible carbohydrates. This situation forces it into a mode of fat burning to produce energy.

Chapter 2
How Long Should It Last?

Many women want to lose weight, but women over the age of 50 are particularly interested in losing weight, boosting their immune system, and having more energy.

If you fit into this group, this phase will address the particular hurdles you may face when doing the Keto diet. For one thing, women in this age range experience slowing metabolisms, making it harder to drop pounds than ever before.

I will cover the tweaks you can make to your Keto diet and lifestyle to accommodate these particular hurdles. I will address any concerns you may have and give you solutions to counteract them.

Women go through menopause sometime between the ages of 45 and 55, and it can be a particularly difficult time. They notice they are putting on weight, and they experience all kinds of unpleasant symptoms such as difficulty sleeping and hot flashes.

But many of these symptoms are temporary. The one that bothers women the most is the one that lasts: weight gain. Women over 50 want to know how they can stave off weight gain and lose the extra pounds they started to put on after menopause.

First of all, I highly recommend intermittent fasting for women in this age group. Intermittent fasting is often paired with Keto for the best possible results in autophagy. Autophagy can be improved through Keto alone, but you don't truly unlock the potential advanced autophagy in your body until you fast between your Ketogenic meals.

The reason I urge you to do intermittent fasting with Keto is that it will help you more with the effects of aging than Keto alone. The autophagy that results from fasting doesn't only help you get better skin, lose weight, and detox your cells—although all these things are worth trying to achieve on their own.

The long-term, anti-aging benefits of intermittent fasting are more important but often ignored. The autophagy that comes from intermittent fasting will help you lower your inflammation, boost your metabolism, enhance your immune system, and more. These are all benefits of autophagy that are backed by scientific research.

Studies show time and time again that fasting works to help women lose weight and improve their health. As a woman over 50, you should consider doing Keto together with fasting.

Scientists are not in agreement about whether menopause itself affects weight. Some say that when women gain weight at this stage in life, it is because of aging alone. They do not believe the hormonal changes from menopause are the reason for the weight gain.

But there is no denying that the lowered estrogen from menopause has some impact on the distribution of fat on the body of a woman over 50. You may have noticed this yourself in your own body: the change in hormones tends to make a woman's fat go from her hips to her waist.

That isn't all, either. Women who go through menopause

also report that they have less energy and have a harder time burning fat. It is no wonder women over 50 want to know how to lose weight. It is such a harder feat at this stage in life.

But don't be misled to believe the change in metabolism is all that is going on here. After all, a doctor studying women over 50 found that women's bodies only metabolized 50 calories fewer calories every day. While this is not a negligible figure, it can hardly be blamed for all of the weight gain that is experienced by women at this age.

You are sure to have experienced some of the other factors that play into weight gain for women at this age. Women over 50 report having more cravings, doing less exercise, and losing more muscle.

As you might guess, many of these factors are related. When you aren't exercising as much, you won't retain as much muscle. If you have more cravings for foods you shouldn't eat, you are more likely to eat those foods and gain weight as a result.

Top it all off with the less efficient metabolisms of women over 50, and it is easy to understand why they have a hard time losing weight. Even if menopause itself isn't the reason women experience this, it all adds up to make weight loss seem impossible, if you don't know anything about Keto or fasting.

Take everything you hear them say about weight gain for women over 50 with a grain of salt. All of us know that it is a reality for women who fall into this age range, but no one knows exactly what the reason for it is. But we do know that Keto and fasting both show fantastic results for these women, so that is the information we should really be paying attention to.

Women in this age range can still go wrong when they try Keto and autophagy, so I have some pieces of advice to give you if you count yourself among this group.

The first piece of advice is to make sure you eat enough protein every day. You might be worried about eating too much protein because you are watching calories, and this is a reasonable thing to do. But when you are on Keto, you need protein as a source of energy.

It is always about balance. On the one hand, you need to make up for the energy you won't be getting from carbs. On the other hand, you have to be careful not to eat too many calories.

As usual, follow along with what your body is telling you. If your body tells you that you still need more energy, wait a bit. You can eat more if some time passes and you still feel hungry.

That probably means you need food for energy. But you have to give yourself this waiting period because otherwise, your mind might be trying to trick you into just eating something you are craving when you are not genuinely hungry.

There is a mental component to this change in diet, too. The problem at the center of women not being able to change their diet is not being used to the real feeling of being full.

By the "real" feeling of being full, I am referring to how people feel when they have eaten enough—not too much.

These days, people eat so many carbs that their idea of fullness is the uncomfortable feeling they have when they eat too many carbs. But you can't lose weight if you see fullness this way. You will consistently overstuff yourself, believing you are making yourself full when you are actually gorging yourself.

To remind yourself what fullness actually feels like, get used to eating without overstuffing yourself. Get used to not feeling uncomfortable after eating. It can feel strangely comforting to be overstuffed with carbs, but that is not a feeling we can let ourselves get used to. If we do, we will never be happy with the simple feeling of fullness.

As I keep emphasizing, we can't villainize fat anymore. The real problem is eating too many calories, most of which tend to come from carbs, not fats. However, women over 50, in particular, need to be careful not to eat too many fats when they follow Keto.

Keto isn't a valid excuse for simply eating a ton of fat. You still need to show some constraint as you do in every diet.

Understanding how to balance your fat consumption will take understanding of how fat fits into Keto. With Keto, you want to be what we call fat-adapted.

You already know what this means; it is just another way of saying what happens in Ketosis. Being fat-adapted means, you are burning fat for energy with Ketones instead of burning glucose with carbs.

I tell you this term because you should eat a lot of healthy fats until you go through significant Ketosis—until you are fat-adapted. Once that happens, you should start being more careful with how much fat you are consuming.

One of the sources women over 50 will get fat from is drinks. Even the drinks you make at home like coffee with milk can be a lot higher in fat than you think. It should go without saying that the specialty coffee you get topped with whipped cream is high in fat.

Women over 50 know they have their own hurdles to

overcome when they chase the goals of weight loss and improved overall health with Keto. But they can do all they can possibly do by following along with the advice in this phase.

Chapter 3
What to Eat?

Cheese and a Healthy Ketogenic Meal

Definition of Cheese

You probably already know that cheese is a dairy product that is obtained from milk. It consists of casein, a milk protein, and can be produced in several distinct flavors. Cheese is made up of protein and fat and is usually from the milk produced by either sheep, goats, buffaloes, or cows. During the production process of cheese, the milk from these animals is acidified. Rennet, a type of enzyme, is added to the acidified milk leading to coagulation. Calcium, fat, protein, and phosphorus are nutrients present in cheese. Cheese is also known for its ability to last for long periods of time life compared to regular milk.

Types of Cheese

There are numerous known brands of cheese across cultures in the world, and because of this, cheese is classified by; method of making and its length of life, texture, animal milk, place of origin, fat content.

Health Benefits of Using Cheese

As stated earlier, cheese is rich in nutrients such as calcium, fat, and iron, which for you on a Keto diet is essential. Similarly, cheese contains zinc, phosphorus, and vitamins; some of the essential requirements for the human body. Cheese, a dairy product, could be better positioned to protect your teeth from cavities.

According to research and study, some types of cheese comprises bits of conjugated linoleic acid, which may help your body against obesity and heart diseases. The calcium in cheese is responsible for strengthening your bones. Cheese, through its containment of vitamin B, is essential in maintaining a healthy and glowing youthful skin.

Risks Associated with the Consumption of Cheese

Cheese does not have fiber, and the ingestion of large amounts could lead to constipation. If you are a lactose-intolerant person, the consumption of cheese could be a challenge for you. This is because cheese comprises lactose, which your body might not be able to digest since it lacks the accountable enzymes for breaking it down. Worry not! Some types of cheese, parmesan, are low in lactose, which might be a benefit if you are a lactose intolerant individual. Casein is a milk protein that you may be sensitive to, and even the low lactose cheese may not be suggested for you.

Recommended Cheese for a Healthy Keto Diet

Mozzarella cheese which contains;

- 5.5g of proteins
- 86 Calories
- 1g of carbs
- 142 mg of calcium
- 6g fat

Feta cheese which contains;

- 4g of fat
- 61 Calories
- 5g of protein
- 1g of carbs
- 59g Calcium

Fruits and Vegetables and a Healthy Ketogenic Meal

What Are Fruits and Vegetables?

Essentially vegetables are plant parts that are eatable by man as food. The parts include stems, seeds, or even flowers. Potatoes and carrots are classified as vegetables since they are edible by human beings. Vegetables are a central part of any meal since they offer vitamins D, B, C, A carbohydrates, and minerals, which are vital for the body in general. Some of the common vegetables worldwide include; potatoes, broccoli, carrots, cabbage (red and green) spinach, legumes, lettuce, onions, and tomatoes.

Fruits are fleshy and frequently the sweet parts of a certain plant that has seeds in them and is edible by man. Human beings across time have depended on fruits as a source of food as well as a way of continuing the growth of plants by replanting the seeds found in the fruits. Most fruits are edible by man in their raw state and may not require any form of cooking before ingesting. Some of the common fruits across cultures in the world include; bananas, oranges, grapes, strawberries, and apples

Fruits and Vegetables That Support the Ketogenic Diet

However, most fruits are high in carbs, and therefore, they are often ignored during a Keto diet plan. However, berries are low in carbs and wealthier in fiber, making them friendly to the Keto diet. Berries (raspberries, strawberries, blackberries, and blueberries) carry antioxidants, which are important in the human body in that they protect you against diseases.

Vegetables are very healthy and are very good for you. If and only if you are on the Keto diet, should you worry about vegetables. As stated in this cook guide, the Keto diet backs a high in fat and low in carb diet plan; you might want to do away with some vegetables that are high in carbs. Carrots and potatoes (sweet potatoes as well as regular potatoes) are high in starch and could possibly interfere with the ketosis process even when ingested in small quantities. Instead, spinach, bell peppers, zucchini, cauliflower, cabbage, broccoli, asparagus, celery, arugula, onion, olives, and pumpkins are all Keto-friendly and thus recommended for your usage.

Why the Ketogenic Fruit and Vegetable Bread?

Any diet rich in fruits and vegetables, the Ketogenic fruit and vegetable bread included, is beneficial to you in that it lowers your chances of suffering from heart diseases. The dietary fiber contained in vegetables is important because it is responsible for the lowering of your body's blood cholesterol levels and reduce your risk of heart diseases. This bread offers you a chance to reduce your chances of developing cardiovascular diseases

This bread also gives you a chance to minimize your chances of coming into contact with cancer. You already know that cancer is deadly, and the mere fact that the bread offers you a shield against cancer should be reason enough for you to bake and consume. The Keto fruit and vegetable bread also lowers your chances of developing prostate cancer if you are a man.

The Keto fruit and vegetable bread also lowers your risk of contracting diabetes.

The fiber in these fruits and vegetable bread is essential in ensuring your digestive system is smooth.

Types of Sweeteners That Support the Keto Diet

As stated earlier in thiscook guidee, ketogenic diets advocate for cutting back in high carbs foods, for example, processed snacks. This is important for you if you want your body to reach the ketosis stage and burn fat instead of carbs to produce energy for your body. Ketosis is also a result of low sugar consumption, which could pose a challenge if you want to sweeten your bread. Lucky for you, there are actually low carb sweeteners that support the Keto diet.

Xylitol - This is a type of sugar alcohol that is usually found in candies, sugar-free gum as well as mints. You may use this sweetener for baking, but you would need more liquids because it tends to increase dryness in the dough as a result of its moisture-absorbent nature. The carbs in this sweetener do not raise your blood sugar levels or insulin levels, unlike the regular sugar.

 Note: Xylitol, when used in high amounts, may cause digestive issues; thus, you should be careful with the amounts you use.

Sucralose - this sweetener passes through your body undigested simply because it is a non-metabolized artificial sweetener that has no carbs or calories, making it popular on the markets since it lacks the bitter test common in many artificial sweeteners.

Stevia – This is a natural sweetener that contains very little amount of carbs or calories. It is from the stevia rebaudiana plant, and unlike the regular sugar, stevia may be useful in lowering blood sugar levels. This sweetener can be found in both the liquids and the powder states, and you could use it to sweeten your food or drinks.

Note: Stevia is much sweeter than regular sugar; thus, you should be careful with the amounts you desire in either your food or drinks or even when using it in a recipe.

Monk fruit sweetener – It is a natural sweetener, and it contains no calories as well as no carbs, which is an essential element in the maintenance of a ketogenic diet. This sweetener is extracted from a plant in China called the monk fruit. The sweetness of this natural sweetener is a result of the natural compounds and sugars, which are antioxidants. This sweetener is essential for regulating blood sugar levels in your body.

Note: You could decide to use the monk fruit sweetener in the place of regular sugar, but you should be in a position to reduce the amount of the sweetener in half in order to achieve the required results.

Why Sweeteners Instead of Regular Sugar?

You might probably be asking yourself this very question. Well, the answer is simple. Sweeteners, like the regular sugar, provide a sweet test during consumption, but what sweeteners have over regular sugar is the ability to not increase the body's blood sugar levels. Extensive conduction of research studies has proven that sweeteners are safe for consumption on a daily basis. For instance, if you are suffering from diabetes, the use of sweetness is useful to you because you do not have to worry about your body's blood sugar levels when you are out enjoying your meals with family and friends.

On a normal diet, human beings consume up to 50% to 55% of carbohydrates. That is more than half the percentage of the whole meal. Proteins take up about 25% of the remaining meal, while fats take up the remaining 20%. This is contrary to the Ketogenic diet, which constitutes about 75% of fats, 20% of protein, and only 5% of carbohydrates. For instance, if you weigh 160 pounds and you are averagely active, then your body would require approximately 30 grams of carbohydrates, 90 grams of protein, and 200 grams of fats for a single day while on the Ketogenic diet.

Cholesterol; is an organic molecule and is important in the structure of the cell membranes. The normal cholesterol levels in an adult are less than 200 mg/dl (milligrams per deciliter). The Ketogenic diet has been reported to regulate the cholesterol levels of some people who adopted the diet. The diet decreases the levels of triglycerides, blood sugar as well as LDL cholesterol.

Protein; it is recommended to ingest between 0.6 – 1.0 grams of protein per pound in the weight of your body (1.6 – 2.0 grams per kilogram). Note that consuming protein in large amounts could get your body out of ketosis.

Fat; the levels of calories originating from fats will depend on how low your consumption of carbohydrates is, and this is probably between 55 – 80%. You could consume;

1,600 calories for about 85 – 130 grams of fat in a day

2,000 calories for about 115 – 170 grams of fat in a day

2,500 calories for about 140 – 210 grams of fat in a day

Carbohydrates; it should be noted that there is no set limit for carbs in a Ketogenic diet. However, anything below 100 grams is considered low carb. You could achieve ketosis is you ate unprocessed real foods.

Sugar; Ketogenic diet ensures you abstain from all foods with carbs, including refined sugar. This means sugar should be limited as low as possible to ensure your body gets into nutritional ketosis.

Grain and dairy; grains and dairy products are rich in carbs, which is against the Ketogenic diet, meaning you have to minimize your consumption to fit in the daily less than 100 grams of carbs.

Chapter 4
How Ketogenic Metabolism Works

Ketosis is a standard metabolic procedure that offers various wellbeing favorable circumstances.

During ketosis, your body changes over fat into mixes known as ketones and begins to utilize them as its essential wellspring of vitality.

Studies have found that consumes fewer calories that energize ketosis are very valuable for weight reduction owing to some degree to hunger suppressant impacts.

Rising examination shows that ketosis may likewise be valuable for, among different conditions, type 2 diabetes and neurological issue.

That being stated, accomplishing ketosis can set aside some effort to work and plan. It's not as simple as cutting carbs.

Here are some productive tips for getting into ketosis.

Reduce Your Carb Consumption

Expending a low carb diet is by a wide margin the most critical factor in achieving ketosis.

Typically, your phones use glucose or sugar as their essential fuel source. In any case, the majority of your cells can likewise utilize different wellsprings of vitality. This includes unsaturated fats, just as ketones, which are otherwise called ketones.

Your body stores glucose in the liver and muscles as glycogen.

At the point when the utilization of starches is extremely little, the glycogen stores decline and the hormone insulin focuses decline. This empowers unsaturated fats to be discharged from your muscle versus fat's shops.

Your liver changes a bit of these unsaturated fats to ketone, acetoacetate and beta-hydroxybutyrate. These ketones can be used as fuel for parts of the cerebrum.

The proportion of carb obstruction required to cause ketosis is somewhat individualized. A couple of individuals need to bind net carbs (complete carbs short fiber) to 20 grams for consistently, while others can accomplish ketosis by eating twice so a great deal or more.

Subsequently, the Atkins diet confirms that carbs should be confined to 20 or fewer grams for consistently for around fourteen days to ensure that ketosis is cultivated.

After this stage, modest quantities of carbs can be familiar with your eating routine a little bit at a time, as long as ketosis is ensured.In a one-week research, people with type 2 diabetes who had limited carb utilization to 21 grams or less every day experienced day by day urinary ketone discharge rates that were multiple times more noteworthy than their standard fixations.

In another exploration, grown-ups with type 2 diabetes were allowed 20–50 grams of edible carbs every day, in light of the number of grams that allowed blood ketone focuses on being kept up inside the objective scope of 0.5–3.0 mmol/L.

These carb and ketone ranges are prescribed for people who need to get ketosis to energize weight reduction, control glucose fixations or lessening hazard factors for coronary illness.

Helpful ketogenic abstains from food utilized for epilepsy or exploratory disease treatment, then again, regularly limit carbs to under 5 percent of calories or under 15 grams for each day to additionally build ketone levels.

Nonetheless, any individual who utilizes an eating regimen for restorative reasons should just do as such under the direction of a clinical expert.

Restricting your starch utilization to 20–50 net grams for every day lessens glucose and insulin fixations, prompting the arrival of putting away unsaturated fats that your liver proselytes to ketones.

Incorporate Coconut Oil In Your Diet

The utilization of coconut oil can help you to get into ketosis.

It incorporates fats called medium-chain triglycerides (MCTs).

In contrast to most fats, MCTs are immediately ingested and taken directly to the liver, where they can be utilized in a split second for vitality or changed to ketones.

As a general rule, it has been proposed that the utilization of coconut oil might be perhaps the most ideal approach to help ketone focuses on people with Alzheimer's ailment and different sensory system diseases.

Despite the fact that coconut oil incorporates four sorts of MCTs, half of its fat is gotten from the sort known as lauric corrosive.

A few examinations propose that fat sources with a more noteworthy extent of lauric corrosive may produce a progressively consistent measure of ketosis. This is on the grounds that it is more continuously used than different MCTs.

MCTs have been utilized to cause ketosis in epileptic children without restricting carbs as definitely as the exemplary ketogenic diet.

In actuality, a few preliminaries have found that a high-MCT diet including 20 percent of starch calories creates impacts tantamount to the great ketogenic diet, which offers under 5 percent of sugar calories.

While adding coconut oil to your eating routine, it's a smart thought to do so gradually to limit stomach related reactions, for example, stomach squeezing or loose bowels.

Start with one teaspoon daily and work up to a few tablespoons every day for seven days. You can find coconut oil in your neighborhood supermarket or get it on the web.

Devouring coconut oil offers your body with MCTs that are quickly retained and changed into ketone bodies by your liver.

Enhance Your Physical Activity

An expanding measure of examination has demonstrated that ketosis can be helpful for certain sorts of athletic execution, including continuance work out.

What's more, being progressively dynamic may help you get into ketosis.

At the point when you practice, your body will be drained from its glycogen shops. Typically, these are renewed when you expend carbs that are separated into glucose and afterward changed to glycogen.

In any case, if the utilization of sugar is limited, the glycogen shops remain little. In response, your liver improves the yield of ketones, which can be utilized as an elective wellspring of vitality for your body.

One examination found that activity improves the rate at which ketones are produced at low blood ketone levels. Be that as it may, when blood ketones are raised, they don't increment with practice and may viably diminish for a short timeframe.

Also, it has been demonstrated that turning out to be in a fasted state is driving up ketone focuses.

In a little examination, nine old females performed either preceding or after a supper. Their blood ketone focuses were 137–314 percent more prominent when utilized before a supper than when utilized after a dinner.

Remember that despite the fact that activity rises ketone yield, it might take one to about a month for your body to acclimate to the utilization of ketones and unsaturated fats as principle energizes. Physical execution might be diminished immediately during this second.

Taking part in physical activity may support ketone fixations during carb restriction. This effect can be improved by working in a quick paced state.

Ramp Up Your Healthy Fat Intake

A lot of good fat can expand your ketone focuses and assist you with accomplishing ketosis.

Indeed, an exceptionally low-carb ketogenic diet limits carbs as well as high in fat.

Ketogenic eats less carbs for weight reduction, metabolic wellbeing and exercise proficiency by and large give between 60-80 percent of fat calories.

The exemplary ketogenic diet utilized for epilepsy is significantly more noteworthy in fat, with commonly 85–90 percent of calories in fat.

Be that as it may, incredibly raised fat utilization doesn't really bring about more prominent ketone focuses.

A three-week exploration of 11 sound individuals differentiated the effects of fasting with particular amounts of fat utilization on ketone centralizations of relaxing.

In general, ketone focuses have been found to be tantamount in people who expend 79% or 90% of fat calories.

Additionally, on the grounds that fat makes up such a major extent of the ketogenic diet, it is fundamental to pick top notch sources.

Extraordinary fats consolidate olive oil, avocado oil, coconut oil, spread, oil and sulfur. Moreover, there are various strong, high-fat sustenances that are in like manner little in carbs.

Nevertheless, if your goal is weight decrease, it's fundamental to guarantee you don't exhaust such countless calories inside and out, as this can make your weight decrease delayed down.

Exhausting on any occasion 60 percent of fat calories will help increase your ketone centers. Pick the extent of sound fats from both animal and plant sources.

Try A Fat Fast Or Short Fast

The other method to get into ketosis is to abandon eating for a couple of hours.

Actually, numerous people have gentle ketosis among lunch and breakfast.

Youngsters with epilepsy now and then quick for 24–48 hours before they start a ketogenic diet. This is accomplished to get into ketosis quickly with the goal that seizures can be diminished all the more quickly.

Irregular fasting, a wholesome technique including intermittent momentary fasting, may likewise cause ketosis.

Likewise, "fat fasting" is another ketone-boosting system that mirrors the effects of fasting.

It incorporates expending around 1,000 calories every day, 85–90 percent of which originate from fat. This blend of low calories and an extremely raised utilization of fat can help you accomplish ketosis quickly.

A 1965 exploration uncovered a significant loss of fat in overweight patients who followed a speedy fat. Be that as it may, different researchers have called attention to that these discoveries seem to have been incredibly misrepresented.

Since fat is so little in protein and calories, a limit of three to five days ought to be followed to evade an inordinate loss of bulk. It might likewise be difficult to adhere to for in excess of a couple of days.

Fasting, irregular fasting and "fat fasting" would all be able to help you get into ketosis relatively quickly.

Maintaining Adequate Protein Intake

Showing up at ketosis needs a protein use that is fitting anyway not over the top.

The commendable ketogenic diet used in epilepsy patients is obliged to increasing ketone centers in both carbs and proteins.

A comparative eating routine may in like manner be

important to infection patients as it would restrain tumor improvement.

In any case, it's definitely not a not too bad practice for the vast majority to decrease proteins to enable ketone to yield.

In any case, it is basic to eat up enough protein to effortlessly the liver with amino acids that can be used for gluconeogenesis, which means' new glucose.' In this strategy, your liver offers glucose to the couple of cells and organs in your body that can't use ketones as fuel.

Chapter 5
The Side Effects of the Ketogenic Diet

The diet can cause a few side effects, including:

Induction Flu: Symptoms include confusion, brain fog, irritability, lethargy, and nausea. These symptoms are common during the first week of the diet.

The cure: consume salt and water. You can cure all these symptoms by getting enough water and salt into your system. Drinking broth daily is a better option.

Leg Cramps: Leg cramps are painful.

The cure: get enough salt and drink plenty of fluids. Taking magnesium supplements is also a good idea. Take three slow-release magnesium tablets daily for the first three weeks.

Constipation: Constipation is another side effect of the diet.

The cure: Getting enough salt and water. Also, include more fiber in your diet, such as fruits and vegetables.

Bad Breath: Bad breath is another unpleasant problem that may arise.

The cure:

Eat more carbohydrates.

Get enough salt and drink enough fluids

Maintain good oral hygiene.

Heart palpitations

The cure: getting enough fluid is the easiest solution

Generally, you can eliminate all the Keto side effects by:

Drinking more water

Increasing salt intake

Eating enough fat

Myths and Misconceptions Concerning the Ketogenic Diet

As one of its side effects, the formation of what is known as ketones is the breaking down of body fat into fatty acids. These acidic fat metabolism by-products tend to increase the level of acidity of the body when they accumulate in the bloodstream and may degenerate into certain conditions of health.

The use of ketogenic diets is one way that ketones can accumulate in the bloodstream. Ketogenic diets such as the famous Atkins Diet are of the view that carbohydrates are the main cause of weight gain and are designed to limit the amount of carbohydrates eaten every day throughout their diets.

Normally, carbohydrates are digested to generate fructose, which is called the body's favorite form of food as it is a quick burning fuel. While the body can metabolize muscle and liver glycogen (a combination of glucose and water) as well as body fat deposits to generate energy, it tends to receive it from high glycemic carbohydrates.

The initial phase of a ketogenic diet usually involves an acute glucose deprivation designed to force the body to exhaust its own available glucose to a significantly lower level that ultimately forces it to switch to burning its fat deposits for energy.

The rate of lipolysis (breakdown of body fat) increases dramatically at this stage of a ketogenic diet to push the body into a state known as ketosis to meet its energy requirements. Ketosis is a condition in which the rate of formation of ketone bodies (by-products of decomposition of fat into fatty acids) is faster than the rate at which the body tissues oxidize them.

Under normal conditions, ketone bodies are easily oxidized to water and carbon dioxide, but their oxidation is very complicated due to increased aggregation during ketosis. The enhanced concentration of ketones in the bloodstream, though, normally leads to increased body acidity causing the body to continue to use water reserves from its cells to flush out the excess ketones.

Therefore, ketogenic diets are designed to achieve two very important weight loss goals: reducing the production of insulin due to the resulting low blood sugar levels; and also the ketosis state which increases the lipolysis rate (fat breakdown). The addition of these two causes allows the use of a ketogenic diet a very successful way to achieve an accelerated loss of weight.

Sadly, the state of elevated ketone aggregation in the skin has been somewhat inconsistent. This is due in part to the fact that many people fail to realize that apart from the ketosis effect of ketogenic diets, another physiological condition may also cause increased accumulation of ketone.

Including ketosis, the other disorder that can induce an elevated concentration of ketones is ketoacidosis. While there is no doubt that both conditions result in increased ketone accumulation and therefore body acidity, the precipitating conditions are very different, however.

Ketoacidosis (also known as Diabetic Ketoacidosis-DKA) is a serious condition in which ketone bodies accumulate in Type I bloodstream diabetics due to the body's inability to produce enough insulin. An increase in counter-regulatory hormones aggravates this condition.

Insulin deficiency in a diabetic contributes to the hyperglycemia-an excessive rise of blood sugar levels that can be as much as four times the bloodstream's usual amount of sugar. When an excessive increase in blood sugar levels happens in a normal individual, the glomeruli of the kidneys remove more insulin than the kidney tubules can reabsorb, resulting in glucose excretion in the urine.

Hyperglycemia is not that dangerous in and of itself, but the side effects can be life-threatening as it usually results in glycosuria (presence of sugar in the urine), excessive urination, and dehydration. Glucose intake of urine is usually associated with exhaustion, nausea, weight loss, and increased appetite.

Continued glucose excretion from the urine and dehydration makes the body seriously hungry for energy. To keep the situation under control, the body can, on the one side, begin to excrete glucose in the urine which triggers a more severe condition, the Hyperosmolar Hyperglycemia Syndrome (HHS), which in people with this condition has a reported mortality rate of around 15%.

On the other hand, as a way to produce more energy to control the situation, the body can begin to break down more triglycerides (stored body fat). Furthermore, this decreased lipolysis (the removal of fatty acids and ketones from fat cells, muscle tissues, and the liver) induces an elevated concentration of ketones (fat degradation by-products) in the urine and the bloodstream to increase blood acidity. What is known as Diabetic Ketoacidosis-DKA is the combination of hyperglycemia and acidosis (abnormal increase in blood acidity).

Thus, while in all cases there is actually a high volume of residual ketones, there is an increased level of blood sugar in the ketoacidosis system. Actually, ketoacidosis can degenerate into hyperventilation, resulting in a subsequent impairment of functions of the central nervous system that can lead to coma and death.

Therefore, it must be stressed that dietitians who use ketogenic diets will ensure that they drink plenty of water to mitigate the elevated acidity rate of the body induced by the release of ketones. This also allows the stored ketones to wash out and preserve a healthy hydration condition.

To sum up, although ketosis is induced by reduced levels of blood sugar, ketoacidosis is caused by increased levels of blood sugar. Although there may be ketone accumulation in both conditions in the bloodstream and urine, their causes are separate poles, however.

Mistake Made on the Keto Diet and How to Overcome Them.

The most common mistakes revolve around food choices. It is important to maintain correct ratios of fats to proteins. The diet program is subject to failure, and poor health may result in failing to maintain the proper amount of fat. The ketogenic diet is based on using fat to burn as fuel in the body. As a result, the body needs fat to burn. Of course, these need to be good fats that promote increases in HDL cholesterol. This will provide good fuel for the body.

It is important to eat the right fats. Margarine, vegetable oil, canola oil, trans fats, and other light non-viscous plant oils and unhealthy fats should be eliminated from the diet. The fat consumed should be high quality like butter from grass-fed animals, olive oil, monounsaturated oils such as from avocados and coconuts. These are oils and fats are the best options for food and keto. The quality of the fat is important so that it is easily processed and converted to fuel.

Be sure to drink adequate amounts of water when you're on the keto diet. Water will help prevent some of the adverse side effects of the keto diet. It can help with constipation and also help dilute ketones, and acids subject accumulate in the bloodstream. Water is an instrumental factor in avoiding additional weight gain from retention and bloating. You will feel better drinking plenty of water.

Failing to drink adequate amounts of water is a common and unhealthy mistake made by ketogenic dieters. Especially at the beginning of the diet, urination will be frequent. The water needs to be replaced, and you may need to replace electrolytes as well. Make sure to feed your body appropriate nutrients.

When you embark on the keto diet, you may find that you eliminate many processed foods from your diet. These foods use salt as a preservative. Because of this, you will need to replace the salt in your system that you will lose as you drink more water and urinate more frequently. This will help you avoid keto flu or reduce the symptoms of the keto flu.

One of the main mistakes people make on the keto diet is eating too many calories.

There is a myth that you can eat whatever you like on the keto diet as long as it is low or no carb and/ or high in fat.

General life principles are still in effect. If you consume more calories than you burn, you'll gain weight. It is important to maintain vigilance in the number of calories consumed and be sure to eat quality foods containing whole grains and fiber. Though there is room in the diet for keto-friendly snacks, try to avoid processed snacks, which may have more carbohydrates than expected. It is important to assess all processed food labels to know the nutritional value of the food you consume.

Chapter 6

The Solution To Your Weight Problems

Routines are very important on this diet, and it's something that will help you stay healthy. As such, in this phase, we are going to be giving you tips and tricks to make this diet work better for you and help you get an idea of routines that you can put in place for yourself.

Tip number one that is so important is DRINK WATER! This is absolutely vital for any diet that you're on, and you need it if not on one as well. However, this vital tip is crucial on a keto diet because when you are eating fewer carbs, you are storing less water, meaning that you are going to get dehydrated very easily. You should aim for more than the daily amount of water however, remember that drinking too much water can be fatal as your kidneys can only handle so much as once. While this has mostly happened to soldiers in the military, it does happen to dieters as well, so it is something to be aware of.

Along with that same tip is to keep your electrolytes. You have three major electrolytes in your body. When you are on a keto diet, your body is reducing the amount of water that you store. It can be flushing out the electrolytes that your body needs as well, and this can make you sick. Some of the ways that you can fight this are by either salting your food or drinking bone broth. You can also eat pickled vegetables.

Eat when you're hungry instead of snacking or eating constantly. This is also going to help, and when you focus on natural foods and health foods, this will help you even more. Eating processed foods is the worst thing you can do for fighting cravings, so you should really get into the routine of trying to eat whole foods instead.

Another routine that you can get into is setting a note somewhere that you can see it that will remind you of why you're doing this in the first place and why it's important to you. Dieting is hard, and you will have moments of weakness where you're wondering why you are doing this. Having a reminder will help you feel better, and it can really help with your perspective.

Tracking progress is something that straddles the fence. A Lot of people say that this helps a lot of people and you can celebrate your wins, however, as everyone is different and they have different goals, progress can be slower in some than others. This can cause others to be frustrated and sad, as well as wanting to give up. One of the most important things to remember is that while progress takes time, and you shouldn't get discouraged if you don't see results right away. With most diets, it takes at least a month to see any results. So don't get discouraged and keep trying if your body is saying that you can. If you can't, then you will need to talk to your doctor and see if something else is for you.

  You should make it a daily routine to try and lower your stress. Stress will not allow you to get into ketosis, which is that state that keto wants to put you in. The reason for this being that stress increases the hormone known as cortisol in your blood, and it will prevent your body from being able to burn fats for energy. This is because your body has too much sugar in your blood. If you're going through a really high period of stress right now in your life, then this diet is not a great idea. Some great ideas for this would be getting into the habit or routine of taking the time to do something relaxing, such as walking and making sure that you're getting enough sleep, leads to another routine that you need to do.

You need to get enough sleep. This is so important not just for your diet but also for your mind and body as well. Poor sleep also raises those stress hormones that can cause issues for you, so you need to get into the routine of getting seven hours of sleep at night on the minimum and nine hours if you can. If you're getting less than this, you need to change the routine you have in place right now and make sure that you establish a new routine where you are getting more sleep. As a result, your health and diet will be better.

Another routine that you need to get into is to give up diet soda and sugar substitutes. This is going to help you with your diet as well because diet soda can actually increase your sugar levels to a bad amount, and most diet sodas contain aspartame. This can be a carcinogen, so it's actually quite dangerous. Another downside is that using these sugar substitutes just makes you want more sugar . Instead, you need to get into the habit of drinking water or sparkling water if you like the carbonation.

Staying consistent is another routine that you need to get yourself into. No matter what you are choosing to do, make sure it's something that you can actually do. Try a routine for a couple of weeks and make serious notes of mental and physical problems that you're going through as well as any emotional issues that come your way. Make changes as necessary until you find something that works well for you and that you can stick to it. Remember that you need to give yourself time to get used to this and time to get used to changes before you give up on them.

Be honest with yourself, as well. This is another big tip for this diet. If you're not honest with yourself, this isn't going to work. Another reason that you need to be honest with yourself is if something isn't working you need to be able to understand that and change it. Are you giving yourself enough time to make changes? Are you pushing too hard? If so, you need to understand what is going on with yourself and how you need to deal with the changes that you're going through. Remember not to get upset or frustrated. This diet takes time, and you need to be able to be a little more patient to make this work effectively.

Getting into the routine of cooking for yourself is also going to help you so much on this diet. Eating out is fun, but honestly, on this diet, it can be hard to eat out. It is possible to do so with a little bit of special ordering and creativity, but you can avoid all the trouble by simply cooking for yourself. It saves time, and it saves a lot of cash.

This another topic falls into both the tip and routine category. Get into the habit of cleaning your kitchen. It's very hard to stick to a diet if your kitchen is dirty and full of junk food. Clear out the junk (donate it if you can, even though it's junk, there are tons of hungry people that would appreciate it) and replace all of the bad food with healthy keto food instead. Many people grab the carbs like crazy because they haven't cleared out their cabinets, and it's everywhere they look. Remember, with this diet, no soda, pasta, bread, candy, and things of that nature. Replacing your food with healthy food and making a regular routine of cleaning your kitchen and keeping the bad food out is going to help you be more successful with your diet, which is what you want here.

Getting into the routine of having snacks on hand is a good idea as well. This keeps you from giving into temptation while you're out, and you can avoid reaching for that junk food. You can make sure that they are healthy, and you will be sticking to your high-intensity diet, which is what you want. There are many different keto snacks that you can use for yourself and to eat. We will have a list of recipes in the following phases to help this as well.

A good tip would be to use keto sticks or a glucose meter. This will give you feedback on whether your users do this diet right. The best option here is a glucose meter. It's expensive, but it's the most accurate. Be aware that if you use ketostix, they are cheaper, but the downside is that they are not accurate enough to help you. A perfect example is that they have a habit of telling people their ketone count is low when they are actually the opposite.

Try not to overeat as this will throw you out of where you need to be. Get into the routine of paying attention to what you're eating and how much. If this is something that you're struggling with, try investing in a food scale. You will be able to see exactly what it is your eating and make sure that your understanding your portions and making sure you stay in ketosis.

Another tip is to make sure that you're improving your gut health. This is so important. Your gut is pretty much linked to every other system in your body, so make sure that this something that you want to take seriously. When you have healthy gut flora, your body's hormones, along with your insulin sensitivity and metabolic flexibility will all be more efficient. When your flexibility is functioning at an optimal level, your body is able to adapt to your diet easier. If it's not, then it will convert the fat your trying to use for energy into body fat.

Batch cooking or meal prepping is another routine that is a good thing to get into. This is an especially good routine for on the go women. When you cook in batches, you are able to make sure that you have meals that are ready to go, and you don't have to cook every single day, and you can save a lot of time as well. You will also be making your environment better for your diet because you're supporting your goals instead of working against them.

The last tip is to mention exercise again. Getting into the routine of exercising can boost your ketone levels, and it can help you with your issues on transitioning to keto. Exercises also use different types of energy for your fuel that you need. When your body gets rid of the glycogen storages, it needs other forms of energy, and it will turn into that energy that you need. Just remember to avoid exercises that are going to hurt you. Stay in the smaller exercises and lower intensity.

Following these tips and getting into these routines is going to help you stay on track and make sure that your diet will go as smoothly as it possibly can.

CHAPTER 7
7-Day Food Program

DAY 1				
Breakfast	**Snack**	**Lunch**	**Snack**	**Dinner**
Scrambled eggs with cheddar cheese, spinach, and sundried tomatoes	Sunflower seeds and mixed nuts	Cauliflower soup with bacon or tofu	Turkey and cucumber roll-ups and celery sticks with guacamole	Garlic and herb shrimp in butter sauce with zucchini noodles

What Do I Eat At Work: Spinach salad with grilled salmon and Melted Cheese

See recipes for lunch and dinner on the following topics.

DAY 2

Breakfast	Snack	Lunch	Snack	Dinner
Fried eggs with sautéed greens and pumpkin seeds	Mixed berries and Macadamia nuts	Chicken salad with cucumber, avocado, tomato, onion, and almonds	Almond milk and chia seed smoothie and berries	Beef stew with mushrooms and onions

What Do I Eat At Work: Tuna salad stuffed in tomatoes

See recipes for lunch and dinner on the following topics.

DAY 3

Breakfast	Snack	Lunch	Snack	Dinner
Almond milk smoothie containing nut butter, spinach, chia seeds, and protein powder	Greek yogurt accompanied with crushed pecans and an almond milk smoothie with greens and protein powder	Chicken tenders served on a bed of greens with cucumbers and goat cheese	Mixed nuts and sliced cheese with olives and bell peppers	Grilled shrimp topped with lemon and served with broccoli

What Do I Eat At Work: Super-Fast Keto Sandwiches

See recipes for lunch and dinner on the following topics

DAY 4

Breakfast	Snack	Lunch	Snack	Dinner
Omelette with mushrooms, bell peppers, and broccoli	Hard-boiled eggs and sliced cheese with sliced bell peppers	Avocado and egg salad served in lettuce cups	Mixed nuts and sliced cheese with olives and bell peppers	Cajun chicken breast with cauliflower rice and Brussels sprouts

What Do I Eat At Work: Slow Cooker Chili with Braised Beef

See recipes for lunch and dinner on the following topics.

DAY 5

Breakfast	Snack	Lunch	Snack	Dinner
Fried eggs with bacon and a side of leafy greens	Walnuts with mixed berries and celery dipped in almond butter	Burger in a lettuce bun, accompanied with avocado and served with a side salad	Celery sticks dipped in almond butter and a handful of mixed berries and nuts	Baked tofu with cauliflower rice, broccoli, bell peppers, and a Thai peanut butter sauce

What Do I Eat At Work: Keto Wraps With Cream Cheese And Salmon

See recipes for lunch and dinner on the following topics.

DAY 6

Breakfast	Snack	Lunch	Snack	Dinner
Baked eggs served in avocado halves	Kale chips and sugar-free jerky (turkey or beef)	Poached salmon and avocado rolls wrapped in seaweed	Kale chips and sliced cheese and olives	Grilled beef kebabs with peppers and broccoli

What Do I Eat At Work: Keto Croque Monsieur

See recipes for lunch and dinner on the following topics.

DAY 7

Breakfast	Snack	Lunch	Snack	Dinner
Scrambled eggs with veggies and salsa	Dried seaweed and cheese slices	Tuna salad made with mayo, served in avocado halves	Sugar-free turkey jerky and an egg and vegetable muffin	Trout broiled with butter and sautéed bok choy

What Do I Eat At Work: Carpaccio

See recipes for lunch and dinner on the following topics.

Chapter 8

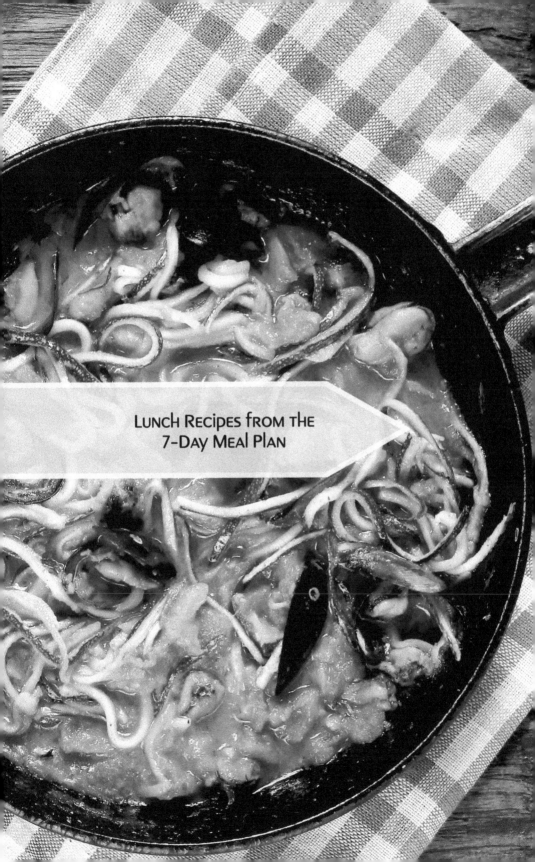

Lunch Recipes from the
7-Day Meal Plan

DAY 1
Cauliflower Soup With
Bacon Or Tofu

PREPARATION

20 MIN

COOKING

60 MIN

SERVES

8

INGREDIENTS

- 1 medium head cauliflower, broken into florets
- 2 Tbsp extra virgin olive oil, divided
- 2 carrots, trimmed and diced
- 3 celery stalks, trimmed and diced
- 2 shallots, trimmed and diced
- 3 garlic cloves, minced
- 1 lb. silken tofu
- 3 Tbsp Kikkoman Traditionally Brewed Soy Sauce
- 8 cups low-sodium chicken or vegetable broth
- For topping (optional):
- Chives, sliced
- Bacon, cooked and crumbled

NUTRITIONS

Calories per serving: 541, Carbohydrates: 4g, Protein: 34g,
Fat: 41g, Sugar: 0.1g, Sodium: 164mg, Fiber: 1.2g

DIRECTIONS

1. Preheat broiler to 425.

2. Line a preparing sheet with tinfoil.

3. Spot cauliflower florets onto the preparing sheet and sprinkle with 1 Tbsp olive oil.

4. Broil cauliflower for around 40 minutes, flipping part of the way through cooking time, or until brilliant earthy colored and delicate. Expel from broiler.

5. In the interim, in an enormous soup pot, heat staying 1 Tbsp olive oil over medium warmth.

6. Include carrots, celery and shallots.

7. Saute for around 5 minutes, mixing regularly, until vegetables perspire and relax however not earthy colored.

8. Include garlic and saute one more moment.

9. Include tofu, separating it in the pot.

10. Include soy sauce and stock.

11. Bring to a stew.

12. When cauliflower is done simmered, add cauliflower to the pot.

13. Heat to the point of boiling, at that point diminish to a stew for 5-10 minutes.

14. Expel pot from heat.

15. Carefully mix soup, utilizing a submersion blender, until smooth.

16. Spoon soup into bowls and top with chives and disintegrated bacon.

17. Present with a warm dried up entire baguette roll.

DAY 2
Chicken Salad With Cucumber, Avocado, Tomato, Onion, And Almonds

PREPARATION
15 MIN

COOKING
15 MIN

SERVES
6

INGREDIENTS

- 1 Rotisserie chicken deboned and shredded (skin on or off)
- 1 large English (or continental) cucumber, halved lengthways and sliced into 1/4-inch thick slices
- 4-5 large Roma tomatoes sliced or chopped
- 1/4 red onion thinly sliced
- 2 avocados peeled, pitted and diced
- 1/2 cup flat leaf parsley chopped*
- 3 tablespoons olive oil
- 2-3 tablespoons lemon juice (or the juice of 2 limes)
- Salt and pepper to taste

Calories per serving: 541, Carbohydrates: 10g, Protein: 40g, Fat: 37g, Sugar: 3g, Sodium: 123mg, Fiber: 6g

DIRECTIONS

1. Mix together shredded chicken, cucumbers, tomatoes, onion, avocados, and chopped parsley in a large salad bowl.

2. Drizzle with the olive oil and lemon juice (or lime juice), and season with salt and pepper. Toss gently to mix all of the flavors through.

DAY 3
Chicken Tenders Served On A Bed Of Greens With Cucumbers And Goat Cheese

PREPARATION

15 MIN

COOKING

10 MIN

SERVES

6

INGREDIENTS

- boneless skinless chicken
- milk
- lemon juice
- sugar
- cornstarch
- pepper
- breadcrumbs
- regular breadcrumbs
- all-purpose flour
- onion powder
- salt or garlic salt
- pepper
- shortening or oil, for frying
- Romaine Lettuce
- Cucumber
- Goat cheese

NUTRITIONS

Calories per serving: 548, Carbohydrates: 3g, Protein: 52g, Fat: 36g, Sugar: 0.1g, Sodium: 175mg, Fiber: 2g

DIRECTIONS

1. Quick marinade to tenderize and flavor chicken.

2. Heat oil for fried chicken tenders

3. Coat the chicken with simple breading

4. Fry the coated chicken tenders until golden brown for 10 minutes

5. On a plate, add rinsed lettuce and chopped cucumber thinly sliced on a half round cut seeds off.

6. Served with goat cheese on top. Enjoy!

DAY 4
Avocado And Egg Salad
Served In Lettuce Cups

PREPARATION

15 MIN

COOKING

15 MIN

SERVES

2

INGREDIENTS

- 1 ripe avocado
- 1 Juice of 1/2 lemon
- 4 hard boiled eggs chilled
- 2 Tablespoons celery
- 1 Tablespoon chopped parsley
- 1/2 teaspoon salt
- 1/4 teaspoon freshly ground pepper
- 1 head buttercrunch lettuce or 4-5 endive bulbs
- 1-2 slices cooked bacon

NUTRITIONS

Calories per serving: 452, Carbohydrates: 2g, Protein: 43g, Fat: 45g, Sugar: 0.1g, Sodium: 155mg, Fiber: 0.7g

DIRECTIONS

1. In a medium bowl, mash avocado and lemon juice together with a fork until it is creamy and smooth. It's okay if there are still a few lumps.

2. With a box grater over the bowl, grate in the four hard boiled eggs. Add the chopped celery, parsley, and seasonings to the bowl .

3. Combine gently with a fork until everything is incorporated. Taste the egg salad and adjust the seasonings as needed. At this point the mixture can be refrigerated for up to 2 hours,

4. Break off the lettuce or endive leaves and arrange them on a plate. Spoon the egg salad into the lettuce cups and top with chopped bacon and more parsley. Serve at once.

DAY 5
Burger In A Lettuce Bun, Accompanied With Avocado And Served With A Side Salad

PREPARATION

15 MIN

COOKING

25 MIN

SERVES

4

INGREDIENTS

Sauce:

- 1/4 cup Greek yogurt
- 2 tablespoons adobo sauce (from canned chipotles in adobo)
- 1 tablespoon Dijon mustard
- 2 dashes Worcestershire sauce

Burgers:

- 2 pounds ground chuck
- 1 teaspoon kosher salt
- 1/2 teaspoon freshly ground black pepper
- 5 dashes Worcestershire sauce

Toppings:

- 1 head iceberg, green leaf or butter lettuce
- 2 avocados, sliced
- 1 tomato, sliced
- 1/4 red onion, thinly sliced into rings
- 12 small sweet pickles, chopped

NUTRITIONS

Calories per serving: 548, Carbohydrates: 2g, Protein: 65g, Fat: 39g, Sugar: 0.1g, Sodium: 175mg, Fiber: 0.7g

DIRECTIONS

1. For the sauce: Mix together the yogurt, adobo sauce, mustard and Worcestershire sauce in a small bowl. Set aside.

2. For the burgers: In a bowl, combine the ground chuck, salt, black pepper and Worcestershire sauce. Form four patties and set aside.

3. Heat a skillet over medium-high heat. Cook the patties until done in the middle, 4 to 6 minutes per side.

4. For the toppings: Cut the base of each lettuce leaf on the head and carefully peel it away so that it stays as intact as possible.

5. Top the patties with avocado slices, tomato slices, red onion rings and chopped pickles, then drizzle with the sauce to taste. Use two or three lettuce leaves per patty and wrap them around the patty as tightly as you can. Slice in half and serve immediately!

DAY 6
Poached Salmon And Avocado Rolls Wrapped In Seaweed

PREPARATION

30 MIN

COOKING

30 MIN

SERVES

2

INGREDIENTS

- 1 to 1½ pounds salmon fillets, pin bones removed
- Salt
- ½ cup dry white wine (a good Sauvignon Blanc)
- ½ cup water
- 1 shallot, peeled and thinly sliced or a few thin slices of onion
- Several sprigs of fresh dill or sprinkle of dried dill
- A sprig of fresh parsley
- Freshly ground black pepper
- A few slices of fresh lemon to serve
- 4 sheets nori seaweed (available from natural food stores and Japanese markets)
- 450 grams (1 pound) cucumbers, thinly sliced with a mandolin slicer (I don't peel my cucumbers; see note)
- toasted sesame seeds
- ground chili powder (optional)
- 1 ripe avocado, sliced into thin wedges
- 100 grams (3 1/2 ounces) tofu, or cooked chicken, or fish (raw and super fresh, or cooked), cut into strips
- long-stem sprouts or sprouted seeds
- soy sauce, for serving

NUTRITIONS

Calories per serving: 584, Carbohydrates: 3g, Protein: 52g, Fat: 45g, Sugar: 0.1g, Sodium: 175mg, Fiber: 3g

DIRECTIONS

1. 1 Sprinkle the salmon fillets with a little salt. Put the wine, water, dill, parsley and shallots or onions in a sauté pan, and bring to a simmer on medium heat.
2. Place salmon fillets, skin-side down on the pan. Cover. Cook 5 to 10 minutes, depending on the thickness of the fillet, or to desired done-ness. Do not overcook.
3. Serve sprinkled with freshly ground black pepper and a slice or two of lemon.
4. Now make the avocado rolls. Have all the ingredients ready and portioned out into four equal servings before you begin, and have a small bowl or glass of water close at hand.
5. Place a sheet of nori on a clean and dry cutting board, shiny side facing down and longest edge facing you.
6. Starting from the left edge, arrange the cucumber slices in overlapping rows on the nori, leaving a 3-cm (1-inch) margin of uncovered nori at right.
7. Sprinkle with sesame and ground chili powder, if using.
8. If using tahini sauce or cashew cheese, drizzle or smear over the cucumber now.
9. If using sliced radishes or salad leaves, arrange in a single layer on top of the cucumber now.
10. Arrange the bulkier fillings -- avocado, tofu, sprouts, herbs, mango, jicama -- in an even, vertical pattern, about 5 cm (2 inches) from the left edge.
11. Rotate the cutting board by a quarter of a turn counter-clockwise so the uncovered strip of nori is furthest from you. Using both hands, start rolling the sheet of nori from the edge closest to you, folding it up and over the fillings, then rolling it snugly away from you (see note).
12. Just as you're about to reach the uncovered strip of nori at the end, dip your fingertips in the bowl of water and dab the nori lightly so it will stick.
13. Set aside, seam side down, and repeat with the remaining ingredients to make three more rolls.
14. Slice into halves or thick slices using a sharp chef knife. Served together with the poached salmon with soy sauce for dipping.

DAY 7
Tuna Salad Made With Mayo, Served In Avocado Halves

PREPARATION

15 MIN

COOKING

0 MIN

SERVES

2

INGREDIENTS

- 1 can (5.5 ounces) water-packed tuna, drained
- 2 tablespoon of mayonnaise
- 2 tablespoon of fresh lemon juice
- 1 chopped celery stalk
- Salt and pepper
- 2 avocados halve and pitted

NUTRITIONS

Calories per serving: 652, Carbohydrates: 1g, Protein: 48g, Fat: 35g, Sugar: 0.1g, Sodium: 145mg, Fiber: 1.5g

DIRECTIONS

1. Combine drained tuna in a small bowl with mayonnaise, lemon juice, and celery. Season with salt and pepper.

2. Fill each avocado with tuna mixture, evenly divided. Garnish with celery leaves if desired.

3. Serve and Enjoy!

Chapter 9

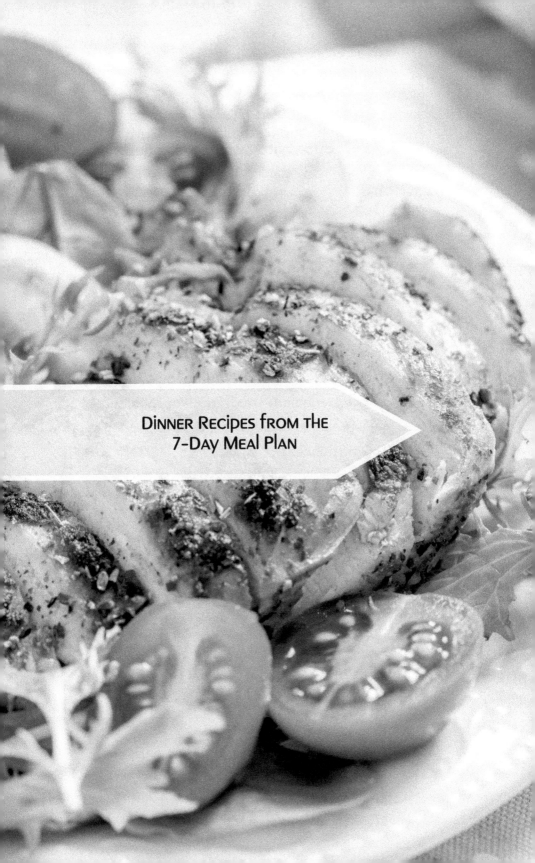

Dinner Recipes from the
7-Day Meal Plan

DAY 1
Garlic And Herb Shrimp In Butter Sauce With Zucchini Noodles

PREPARATION

15 MIN

COOKING

30 MIN

SERVES

6

INGREDIENTS

- 4 tablespoons unsalted butter, divided
- 4 cloves garlic, minced and divided
- 1 pound (3 medium-sized) zucchini, spiralized*
- Kosher salt and freshly ground black pepper, to taste
- 1 shallot, minced
- 1 pound medium shrimp, peeled and deveined
- 2 teaspoons lemon zest
- 2 tablespoons chopped fresh parsley leaves

NUTRITIONS

Calories per serving: 352, Carbohydrates: 2g, Protein: 42.5g, Fat: 42g, Sugar: 0.1g, Sodium: 152mg, Fiber: 0.7g

DIRECTIONS

1. Melt 1 tablespoon butter in a large skillet over medium heat. Add 2 cloves garlic and cook, stirring frequently, until fragrant, about 1 minute.

2. Stir in zucchini noodles until just tender, about 2-3 minutes; season with salt and pepper, to taste. Set aside and keep warm.

3. Melt the remaining 3 tablespoons butter in the skillet. Add remaining 2 cloves garlic and shallot, and cook, stirring frequently, until fragrant, about 2 minutes.

4. Add shrimp; season with salt and pepper, to taste. Cook, stirring occasionally, until pink and cooked through, about 3-4 minutes. Stir in lemon zest and parsley.

5. Serve immediately with zucchini noodles.

DAY 2
Beef Stew With Mushrooms And Onions

PREPARATION

15 MIN

COOKING

30 MIN

SERVES

6

INGREDIENTS

- 2 lbs. beef sirloin or chuck cut into cubes
- 1 1/2 teaspoons sea salt
- 1/4 teaspoon ground black pepper
- 1/4 cup butter
- 2 lbs. chopped white mushrooms
- 1 medium yellow onion chopped
- 5 cloves garlic crushed
- 1/4 cup tomato paste
- 1 can 10 oz. cream of mushroom
- 4 cups beef broth
- 2 teaspoons dried parsley flakes
- 1/2 teaspoon dried oregano

NUTRITIONS

Calories per serving: 452, Carbohydrates: 2g, Protein: 49g, Fat: 44g, Sugar: 2g, Sodium: 174mg, Fiber: 3g

DIRECTIONS

1. Rub salt and ground black pepper on the beef. Let it stay for 10 minutes.

2. Melt 1 tablespoon butter in a Dutch oven or cooking pot. Put the beef in and cook for 3 to 5 minutes or until the color turns light brown.

3. Remove the beef. Set Aside. Melt the remaining butter in the same cooking pot.

4. Once the butter melts, sauté the mushrooms, onions, and garlic. Continue to cook until the mushrooms become soft.

5. Add the beef. Cook for 2 minutes.

6. Add the tomato paste, parsley, oregano, and beef broth. Stir and let boil. Cover and simmer 60 min.

7. Add the cream of mushroom. Stir and cook for 2 to 3 minutes.

8. Turn the heat off. Transfer to a serving plate. Share and enjoy!

DAY 3
Grilled Shrimp Topped With Lemon And Served With Broccoli

PREPARATION

15 MIN

COOKING

30 MIN

SERVES

6

INGREDIENTS

- 2 large heads broccoli, trimmed into bite-sized florets
- 4 tablespoons olive oil, divided
- 1 teaspoon kosher salt, plus more to taste if desired
- 1 teaspoon freshly ground black pepper, plus more to taste if desired
- 1 pound raw shrimp, cleaned, deveined, shells removed (I used U12 shrimp, i.e. 12 per 1 pound)
- 1/4 cup unsalted butter, melted
- 1/4 cup freshly squeezed lemon juice

NUTRITIONS

Calories per serving: 425, Carbohydrates: 6g, Protein: 47g, Fat: 32g, Sugar: 0.1g, Sodium: 162mg, Fiber: 0.7g

DIRECTIONS

1. Preheat oven to high broiler setting and place the top oven rack about 4 inches below the broiler. Line a half-sheet pan with aluminum foil for easier cleanup, add the broccoli, evenly drizzle with 2 tablespoons olive oil, 1 teaspoon salt, 1 teaspoon pepper, toss with your hands to combine, place sheet pan under the broiler, and broil for about 5 minutes, or until florets are turning lightly browned and dried out looking on the tips of the florets.

2. Remove pan from the oven, flip and toss the broccoli, add the shrimp, evenly drizzle the shrimp with the remaining 2 teaspoons olive oil, and return pan to the broiler for about 2 to 3 minutes, or until shrimp are cooked through. There is no need to flip them. Remove pan from the oven and set aside.

3. Melt the butter in a small microwave-safe bowl, add the lemon juice, stir to combine, and evenly drizzle over the shrimp and broccoli, as desired. Taste and check for seasoning balance and add more salt and/or pepper, as desired, and serve immediately. Recipe will keep airtight in the fridge for up to 3 days.

DAY 4
Cajun Chicken Breast With Cauliflower Rice And Brussels Sprouts

PREPARATION

15 MIN

COOKING

40 MIN

SERVES

3

INGREDIENTS

- ¼ lb. Chicken Breast
- 1 tablespoon avocado oil or olive oil
- 1 small onion, diced
- 3 cloves garlic, minced
- 8 cups riced cauliflower
- 1 cup chicken stock
- 1 tablespoon plus 2 teaspoons Creole seasoning, more to taste
- 1 small red bell pepper, diced
- 1 small green bell pepper, diced
- 1 small yellow bell pepper, diced
- chopped fresh flat-leaf parsley, for garnish
- 5 ounces Brussel Sprouts

NUTRITIONS

Calories per serving: 475, Carbohydrates: 2g, Protein: 45g, Fat: 35g, Sugar: 0.1g, Sodium: 172mg, Fiber: 4g

DIRECTIONS

1. Heat the oil in a large skillet over medium heat.

2. Season strips of chicken breasts with salt and pepper.

3. Pan fry for 3mins each side or until cooked. Then set aside.

4. On the same pan, add the onion and garlic and sauté until the onions are translucent and the garlic is fragrant.

5. Add the cauliflower, and sauté until the cauliflower is tender, about 15 minutes.

6. Add the stock and the seasoning and cook, stirring often, for an additional 10 to 15 minutes, or until all of the stock is evaporated and the rice is tender but not mushy.

7. Add the bell peppers and cook an additional 10 minutes.

8. Blanch Brussel sprouts by boiling water for 5 minutes, followed by an ice bath.

9. Sauté with garlic and onion. Add fresh lemon juice, Balsamic vinegar and toss so Brussels sprouts are evenly coated or sprinkle with Parmesan cheese.

10. Add chopped Brussels sprouts to the dish.

11. Garnish with parsley before serving.

DAY 5
Baked Tofu With Cauliflower Rice, Broccoli, Bell Peppers, And A Thai Peanut

PREPARATION
15 MIN

COOKING
45 MIN

SERVES
4

INGREDIENTS

- 12 ounces extra-firm tofu
- 1 tbsp toasted sesame oil
- 1 small head cauliflower
- 2 cloves garlic
- 1 1/2 tbsp toasted sesame oil
- 1/4 cup low sodium soy sauce
- 1/4 cup light brown sugar
- 1/2 tsp chili garlic sauce
- 2 1/2 tbsp peanut butter or almond butter

Veggies:

- baby bok choy, green onion, red pepper, broccoli

Toppings:

- fresh lime juice, cilantro, sriracha

NUTRITIONS

Calories per serving: 416, Carbohydrates: 6g, Protein: 47g, Fat: 32g, Sugar: 0.1g, Sodium: 162mg, Fiber: 9g

DIRECTIONS

1. Begin by draining tofu 1.5 hours before you want your meal ready. If your block of tofu is larger than 12 ounces, trim it down. You don't need a full pound for this recipe.

2. Roll tofu in an absorbent towel several times and then place something heavy on top to press. I use a pot on top of a cutting board and sometimes add something to the pot to add more weight. Do this for 15 minutes.

3. Near the end of draining, preheat oven to 400 degrees F (204 C) and cube tofu. Place on a parchment-lined baking sheet and arrange in a single layer. Bake for 25 minutes to dry/firm the tofu. Once baked, remove from oven and let cool.

4. Prepare sauce by whisking together ingredients until combined. Taste and adjust flavor as needed. I often add a little more sweetener and peanut butter.

5. Add cooled tofu to the sauce and stir to coat. Let marinate for at least 15 minutes to saturate the tofu and infuse the flavor.

6. In the meantime, shred your cauliflower into rice by using a large grater or food processor. You don't want it too fine, just somewhat close to the texture of rice. Set aside. Mince garlic if you haven't already done so, and prepare any veggies you want to add to the dish.

7. Heat a large skillet over medium to medium-high heat and if adding any veggies to your dish, cook them now in a bit of sesame oil and a dash of soy sauce. Remove from pan and set aside and cover to keep warm.

8. Use a slotted spoon to spoon tofu into the preheated pan. Add a few spoonful's of the sauce to coat. Cook, stirring frequently for a few minutes until browned. It will stick to the pan a bit, so don't worry. Remove from pan and set aside and cover to keep warm.

9. Rinse your pan under very hot water and scrape away any residue. Place back on oven.

10. Add a drizzle of sesame oil to the pan, then add garlic and cauliflower rice and stir. Put cover on to steam the "rice." Cook for about 5-8 minutes until slightly browned and tender, stirring occasionally. Then add a few spoonful's of sauce to season and stir.

11. Place cauliflower rice and top with veggies and tofu. Serve with any leftover sauce. Leftovers reheat well and will keep covered in the fridge for up to a couple days.

DAY 6
Grilled Beef Kebabs With Peppers And Broccoli

PREPARATION
20 MIN

COOKING
35 MIN

SERVES
4

INGREDIENTS

- 1/3 c. low-sodium soy sauce
- 1/4 c. brown sugar
- Juice of 2 limes (or 1 if large), plus more for serving
- 1 tbsp. ground ginger
- 1 lb. sirloin steak, cut into cubes
- 2 c. broccoli florets
- 2 tbsp. extra-virgin olive oil
- Freshly ground black pepper
- Green onions, for garnish

NUTRITIONS

Calories per serving: 321, Carbohydrates: 3g, Protein: 53g, Fat: 25g, Sugar: 0.1g, Sodium: 132mg, Fiber: 3g

DIRECTIONS

1. Heat grill to medium-high. In a small bowl, whisk together soy sauce, brown sugar, lime juice and ginger.

2. Add steak and toss until coated. Let marinate in the fridge, at least 15 minutes and up 2 hours.

3. In another bowl, toss broccoli florets with olive oil.

4. Skewer steak and broccoli and season all over with pepper.

5. Grill, turning occasionally, until steak is medium, 8 minutes.

6. Squeeze with lime, garnish with green onions, and serve.

DAY 7
Trout Broiled With Butter And Sautéed Bok Choy

PREPARATION
15 MIN

COOKING
30 MIN

SERVES
6

INGREDIENTS

- 1/2 tablespoon honey
- 1 tablespoon tamari
- 1 large garlic clove, minced
- 3/4 teaspoon chili powder
- 1 filet (6 ounce) trout fish (skin on)
- Sea salt, to taste
- Fresh ground black pepper to taste
- 2 heads baby bok choy, rinsed and halved
- 1/2 teaspoon sesame oil
- 1/4 teaspoon hot pepper flakes

Calories per serving: 352, Carbohydrates: 2g, Protein: 42.5g, Fat: 42g, Sugar: 0.1g, Sodium: 152mg, Fiber: 0.7g

DIRECTIONS

1. Preheat oven to 425 degrees Fahrenheit and line a baking sheet with parchment paper.

2. In a bowl, whisk together the honey, half the tamari, minced garlic and chili powder; stir well to mix.

3. Lay the rainbow trout skin side down onto parchment paper and season with salt and pepper. Use a brush to spread the honey garlic mixture onto the fish.

4. Add the bok choy to a large mixing bowl and drizzle with the remaining tamari and sesame oil. Toss well.

5. Transfer bok choy to baking sheet and organize it around the rainbow trout.

6. Place in the oven and bake for 12 to 15 minutes or until the fish flakes easily when poked with a fork.

7. Remove from oven and enjoy.

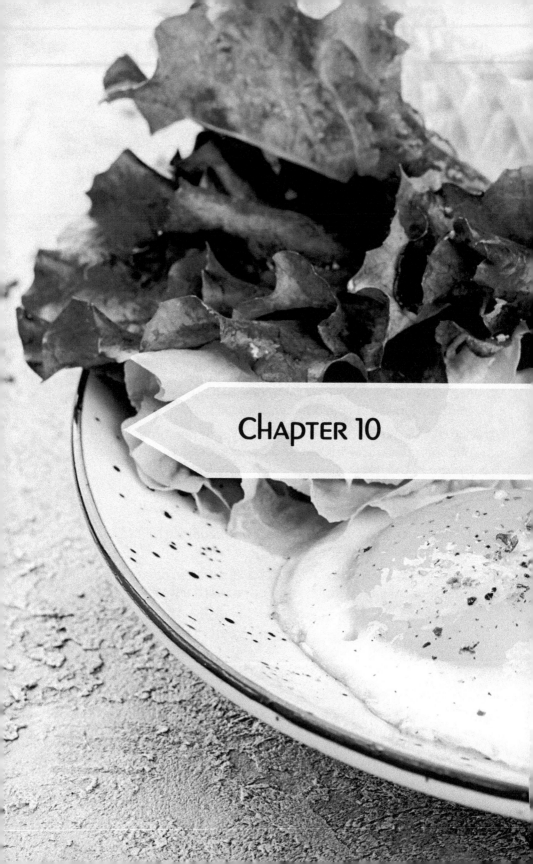

Chapter 10

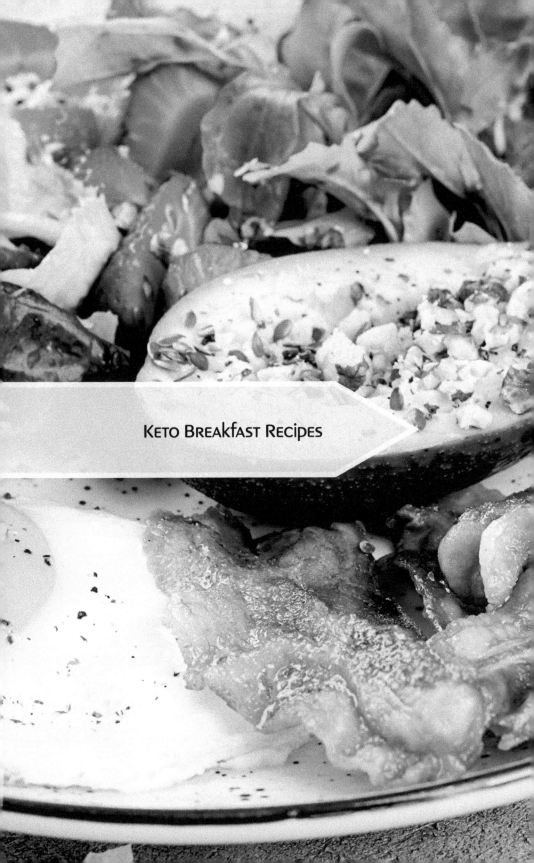

Keto Breakfast Recipes

1. Biscuits and Gravy

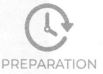

PREPARATION

15 MIN

COOKING

60 MIN

SERVES

6

INGREDIENTS

- ¼ tsp. sea salt
- ¼ tsp. xanthan gum*
- ½ tsp. garlic powder
- 1 tbsp. baking powder
- 2 lg. eggs
- 3 c. almond flour, finely ground
- 6 tbsp. butter softened
- ¼ tsp. xanthan gum*
- ½ c. chicken broth
- ½ c. heavy whipping cream
- ½ tsp. black pepper, ground
- ½ tsp. sea salt
- 1 lb. ground breakfast sausage
- 2 oz. cream cheese
- 2 tbsp. butter

NUTRITIONS

Calories per serving: 521, Carbohydrates: 5g, Protein: 42g,
Fat: 46g, Sugar: 0.1g, Sodium: 165mg, Fiber: 0.7g

DIRECTIONS

1. Preheat the oven to 400° Fahrenheit and line a baking sheet with parchment paper.

2. In a large mixing bowl, combine all the dry ingredients Directions: biscuits and whisk together.

3. Add softened butter and the eggs to the dry ingredients and whisk until completely mixed.

4. Gently form the dough into 10 biscuit shapes with your hands and place them one to two inches apart on the baking sheet.

5. Bake for 12 to 14 minutes, just until the tops begin to take on a golden brown color.

6. Let cool completely.

7. Warm a skillet over medium heat and brown the breakfast sausage completely, breaking it up into smaller pieces as you do so.

8. Add the butter and cream cheese to the skillet and stir until completely combined. This could take a few minutes to reach an even texture.

9. Add the cream and broth to the pan and continue to mix, then add the xanthan gum, salt, and pepper and mix once more.

10. Heat the mixture until it reaches a low boil, then kill the heat. Stir with the heat off until it starts to thicken into a gravy.

11. Serve warm over the biscuits!

* This is used to thicken the stew but can be substituted for arrowroot, cornstarch, or flour. Chef's choice!

2. Banana Nut Muffins

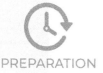
PREPARATION
15 MIN

COOKING
20 MIN

SERVES
7

INGREDIENTS

- ¼ c. almond flour
- ¼ c. almond milk, unsweetened
- ¼ c. sour cream
- ½ c. erythritol, or equal measure of preferred sweetener
- ½ tsp. cinnamon, ground
- 1 tsp. vanilla extract
- 2 ½ tsp. banana extract
- 2 lg. eggs
- 2 tbsp. flaxseed, ground
- 2 tsp. baking powder
- 5 tbsp. butter, melted

NUTRITIONS

Calories per serving: 545, Carbohydrates: 2g, Protein: 47g, Fat: 34g, Sugar: 0.1g, Sodium: 175mg, Fiber: 0.7g

DIRECTIONS

1. ¾ c. walnuts, chopped

2. 1 tbsp. almond flour

3. 1 tbsp. butter, chilled and cubed

4. 1 tbsp. erythritol, powdered, or equal measure of preferred powdered sweetener.

5. Preheat the oven to 350° Fahrenheit and fill a muffin tin with muffin liners.

6. In a large mixing bowl, combine sweetener, almond flour, flaxseed, cinnamon, and baking powder. Whisk until completely combined.

7. Stir in the melted butter, extracts, almond milk, and sour cream. Add the eggs to the mixture and mix until completely combined.

8. Fill each tin about ¾ of the way and set aside.

9. Combine nuts, almond flour, and butter in the food processor and pulse until the nuts are chopped into small pieces. If the mixture seems a little too dry, you may add more butter to moisten it.

10. Sprinkle the mixture evenly over the tops of all the muffin tins.

11. Sprinkle the sweetener over each muffin.

12. Bake for 20 minutes, or until they've taken on a golden brown color and an inserted toothpick comes out clean.

13. Let cool for 30 minutes or more to cool and firm.

14. Enjoy!

3. Egg Cups with Mushrooms

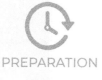

PREPARATION
15 MIN

COOKING
20 MIN

SERVES
5

INGREDIENTS

- ¼ c. almond milk, unsweetened
- 1/3 c. feta cheese crumbles
- ½ tbsp. extra virgin olive oil
- 10 slices bacon
- 2 cloves garlic, minced
- 3 c. baby leaf spinach
- 6 lg. eggs
- 8 oz. mushrooms, sliced
- Sea salt & pepper, to taste

NUTRITIONS

Calories per serving: 512, Carbohydrates: 2g, Protein: 45g,
Fat: 41g, Sugar: 0.1g, Sodium: 178mg, Fiber: 0.7g

DIRECTIONS

1. Preheat the oven to 400° Fahrenheit and line 10 wells of a muffin tin with a slice of bacon, pressing it gently to the sides. You'll notice some overlapping, which is perfectly fine.

2. Bake for 15 minutes to allow it to partially cook.

3. Heat a large skillet over medium heat and warm the olive oil in it. Once warm, add the mushrooms and garlic, sautéing them for about five minutes.

4. Once the mushrooms gain a bit of color, add the spinach into the pan and stir to wilt it, then set aside off the burner.

5. In a mixing bowl, combine the eggs, almond milk, and salt & pepper. Whisk until completely combined and pull the muffin tin out of the oven.

6. You may find that you have excess grease to dispose of from the muffin tin. You can soak up the grease with a paper towel, or you can pull the bacon out of the wells, turn it upside down to drain, then set the bacon back into the cups. If you decide to completely wipe out the grease from the pan, spritz it with a little non-stick spray before putting the bacon back into the tin.

7. Evenly put the veggies into each tin, then pour the egg mixture over top of it to fill each one most of the way.

8. Bake for 15 to 20 minutes, or until the tops are golden.

9. Cool for about five minutes before freeing the cups from the tin by running a butter knife along the edges gently.

4. Green Smoothie

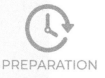

PREPARATION	COOKING	SERVES
15 MIN	0 MIN	6

INGREDIENTS

- 1 ½ c. ice
- 1 med. banana
- 2 handfuls baby leaf spinach
- ½ avocado
- 1 ½ c. almond milk, unsweetened
- 2 scoops protein powder

NUTRITIONS

Calories per serving: 452, Carbohydrates: 2g, Protein: 43g, Fat: 45g, Sugar: 0.1g, Sodium: 155mg, Fiber: 0.7g

DIRECTIONS

1. Combine all ingredients into a blender.
2. Blend until very smooth.
3. Serve chilled and enjoy!

5. Coconut Pancakes

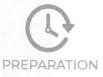

PREPARATION
15 MIN

COOKING
20 MIN

SERVES
5

INGREDIENTS

- 1/8 tsp. sea salt
- ¼ c. coconut flour
- 1 tsp. baking powder
- 1 tsp. vanilla extract
- 2 tbsp. extra virgin olive oil
- 2 tbsp. maple syrup
- 3 lg. eggs

Calories per serving: 352, Carbohydrates: 2g, Protein: 42.5g, Fat: 42g, Sugar: 0.1g, Sodium: 152mg, Fiber: 0.7g

DIRECTIONS

1. In a large mixing bowl, combine coconut flour, olive oil, eggs, maple syrup, vanilla extract, salt, and baking powder. Stir thoroughly using a whisk and break up any clumps as you go.

2. Heat a skillet over medium heat and grease it using more olive oil or your preferred fat source.

3. Spoon the batter into the skillet about ¼ cup at a time and allow to cook for about four to five minutes until bubbles form in the center of the pancake, then flip and cook for another four to five minutes.

4. Repeat until you're out of batter and serve warm!

6. Spinach Artichoke Breakfast Bake

PREPARATION
15 MIN

COOKING
20 MIN

SERVES
7

INGREDIENTS

- ¼ c. milk, fat-free
- ¼ tsp. ground pepper
- 1/3 c. red pepper, diced
- ½ c. feta cheese crumbles
- ½ c. scallions, finely sliced
- ¾ c. canned artichokes, chopped, drained, & patted dry
- 1 ¼ tsp. kosher salt
- 1 clove garlic, minced
- 1 tbsp. dill, chopped
- 10 oz. spinach, frozen, chopped & drained
- 2 tbsp. parmesan cheese, grated
- 4 lg. egg whites
- 8 lg. eggs

NUTRITIONS

Calories per serving: 574, Carbohydrates: 2g, Protein: 47g, Fat: 54g, Sugar: 0.1g, Sodium: 254mg, Fiber: 0.7g

DIRECTIONS

1. Preheat the oven to 375° Fahrenheit and grease a large baking dish with nonstick spray or preferred fat source.

2. In a small bowl, combine the spinach, artichoke, scallions, garlic, red pepper, and fill. Combine completely and then pour into the baking dish, spreading into an even layer.

3. In a mixing bowl, combine eggs, egg whites, salt, pepper, parmesan, and milk. Whisk until completely combined, then add feta and mix once more.

4. Pour the egg mixture evenly over the vegetables in the baking dish.

5. Bake for about 35 minutes, until a butter knife inserted in the center comes out clean.

6. Allow to cool for about 10 minutes before cutting into eight equal pieces.

7. Serve warm!

7. Granola Bars

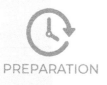

PREPARATION
15 MIN

COOKING
20 MIN

SERVES
6

INGREDIENTS

- 2 c. almonds, chopped
- ½ c. pumpkin seeds, raw
- 1/3 c. coconut flakes, unsweetened
- 2 tbsp. hemp seeds
- ¼ c. clear Sukrin Fiber Syrup
- ¼ c. almond butter
- ¼ c. erythritol, powdered, or equal measure of preferred sweetener
- 2 tsp. vanilla extract
- 1/2 tsp. sea salt

NUTRITIONS

Calories per serving: 254, Carbohydrates: 2g, Protein: 42.5g, Fat: 47g, Sugar: 0.1g, Sodium: 145mg, Fiber: 0.7g

DIRECTIONS

1. Line a small, square baking dish with parchment paper.

2. In a mixing bowl, combine almonds, pumpkin seeds, coconut flakes, and hemp seeds. Stir until evenly mixed.

3. Over medium heat, combine the syrup, almond butter, sweetener, and salt and stir until it's smooth and easy to pull the spoon through.

4. Remove the pan from the heat and stir the vanilla extract into the mixture.

5. Pour the syrup over the seeds and stir completely.

6. Pour the mixture into the baking dish and press evenly into one layer and press until the top is even.

7. Let cool completely and slice into 12 bars.

8. Banana Bread

PREPARATION
15 MIN

COOKING
20 MIN

SERVES
7

INGREDIENTS

- ¼ c. almond milk, unsweetened
- ¼ c. coconut flour
- ¼ tsp. sea salt
- ½ c. erythritol, or equal measure of preferred sweetener
- ½ c. walnuts, chopped
- ½ tsp. xanthan gum*
- 2 c. almond flour
- 2 tsp. baking powder
- 2 tsp. banana extract
- 2 tsp. cinnamon, ground
- 4 lg. eggs
- 6 tbsp. butter softened

Calories per serving: 245, Carbohydrates: 4g, Protein: 47g, Fat: 22g, Sugar: 2g, Sodium: 125mg, Fiber: 0.7g

DIRECTIONS

1. Preheat the oven to 350° Fahrenheit and line a loaf pan with parchment paper.

2. In a large mixing bowl, combine the flours, baking powder, sea salt, and cinnamon and mix thoroughly.

3. In another bowl, cream the butter and the sweetener with a hand mixer. Beat the eggs into the mixture and then do the same with both the vanilla and the banana extracts.

4. Pour the dry ingredients into the wet and mix on low with your hand or stand mixer until a batter begins to form.

5. Mix the chopped walnuts into the mixture.

6. Pour the batter into the loaf pan and sprinkle more walnuts onto the top.

7. Bake for about an hour, or until the top is slightly golden and an inserted toothpick comes out clean.

8. Allow to cool completely before slicing into 12 pieces.

9. Serve!

*This is used to thicken the stew but can be substituted for arrowroot, cornstarch, or flour. Chef's choice!

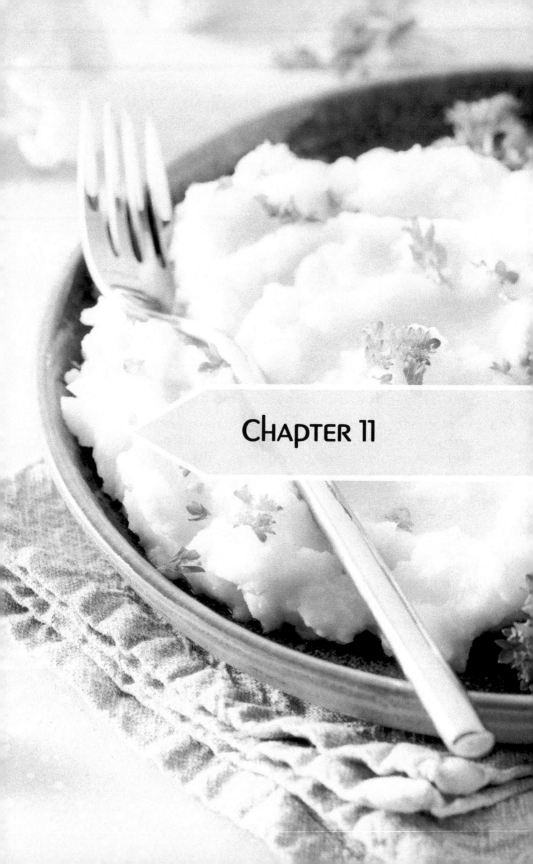

Chapter 11

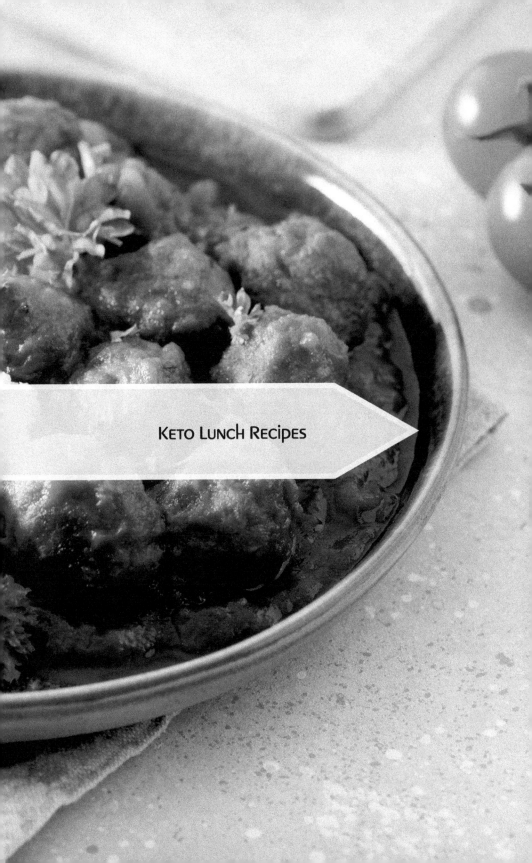

Keto Lunch Recipes

9. Carpaccio

PREPARATION

10 MIN

COOKING

10 MIN

SERVES

2

INGREDIENTS

- 100 grams of smoked prime rib
- 30 grams of arugula
- 20 grams of Parmesan cheese
- 10 grams of pine nuts
- 7 grams of butter
- 3 tablespoons of olive oil with orange
- 1 tablespoon of lemon juice
- Pepper and salt

NUTRITIONS

Calories: 350 kcal, Gross carbohydrates: 3 g ,Protein: 31 g,
Fat: 24 g, Fiber: 1 g, Net carbohydrates: 2 g,
Macro fat: 42 %, Macro proteins: 54 %,
Macro carbohydrates: 4 %

DIRECTIONS

1. Arrange the meat slices on a plate.

2. Place meat products on a plate

3. Wash the arugula and pat dry or use a salad spinner.

4. Place the arugula on top of the meat.

5. Place arugula on the meat

6. Scrape some curls from the Parmesan cheese and spread them over the arugula.

7. Spread Parmesan cheese over the arugula

8. Put the butter in a small frying pan. Add the pine nuts as soon as the butter has melted. Let the pine nuts bake for a few minutes over a medium heat and then sprinkle them over the carpaccio.

9. Sprinkle pine nuts over the carpaccio

10. Make vinaigrette by mixing the lemon juice into the olive oil. Season with pepper and salt and drizzle over the carpaccio.

10. Keto Spring Frittata

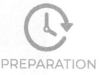

PREPARATION

5 MIN

COOKING

10 MIN

SERVES

2

INGREDIENTS

- 1 zucchini
- 0.5 bunch of mint
- 6 eggs
- pinch of cayenne pepper
- 1 sprig of thyme or 1 teaspoon of dried thyme
- 80 grams of Pecorino cheese
- 0.5 red chili pepper
- 100 grams of feta cheese
- 3 tablespoons of extra virgin olive oil
- 0.25 teaspoon truffle oil optional
- Salt to taste
- Salad
- 50 grams of watercress
- 0.5 stalk of celery
- 75 grams of fresh (raw) peas still in the pod
- 1 tablespoon of lemon juice
- 2 tablespoons of extra virgin olive oil
- Herb cheese or boursin
- 200 grams of herb cheese or boursin

NUTRITIONS

Calories: 955 kcal, Gross carbohydrates: 16 g, Protein: 46 g,
Fats: 78 g, Fiber: 2 g, Net carbohydrates: 14 g, Macro fats: 57 %,
Macro proteins: 33 %, Macro carbohydrates: 10 %

DIRECTIONS

1. If you have an oven with a grill, turn the grill on at the highest setting.
2. Grate the zucchini by hand or in the food processor and put in a bowl. Sprinkle some salt over the grated zucchini.
3. Put the zucchini in a strainer and press the zucchini firmly so that some of the moisture goes out.
4. Wash the mint and pat dry. Remove the leaves from the twigs and cut them into pieces. Add to the zucchini and mix together.
5. Heat the olive oil in a small (frying) pan over a medium-high heat. Add the zucchini as soon as the oil is hot and spread over the pan. Lower the heat to moderate.
6. Spread the zucchini over the pan
7. Beat the eggs in the bowl and add the truffle oil, cayenne pepper and thyme leaves. Grate the pecorino and add half of the pecorino to the bowl.
8. Beat eggs with thyme and cayenne pepper and truffle oil
9. Pour the beaten eggs over the zucchini in the frying pan. Mix in the zucchini. Reduce the heat and simmer for 5 minutes while making the salad.
10. Put the frittata in a baking dish or on a large plate and sprinkle the rest of the pecorino over it. Place as high as possible in the oven, just below the grill and brown for 5 minutes. If you don't have a grill, let the frittata cook on the stove for 5 minutes with a lid on the pan, if you want the cheese to melt, you can gently turn the frittata by putting a lid or plate on the pan and then turning it over.
11. Spring frittata under the grill
12. Wash the chili pepper and remove the seeds. Cut into small rings and sprinkle over the frittata as soon as it comes out of the oven. Also crumble the feta over the frittata.
13. Spring frittata from Jamie Oliver
14. Salad
15. Bring a saucepan of water to the boil and add a pinch of salt.
16. Wash the watercress and pat dry. Put in a salad bowl. Wash the celery and cut into 5 cm pieces and cut them into thin sticks (also use the celery leaves).
17. Remove the peas from the cap and blanch them for 1-2 minutes in the boiling water in the saucepan (the same applies to frozen peas or snow peas). Then let them drain in a colander. If you have fresh peas from the pod, this is not necessary.
18. While the peas are cooling down, make vinaigrette by mixing lemon juice with the extra virgin olive oil.
19. Add the peas to the salad and pour the vinaigrette over it. Mix everything together very well.

11. Super-Fast Keto Sandwiches

PREPARATION
5 MIN

COOKING
5 MIN

SERVES
1

INGREDIENTS

- 1 teaspoon of hemp flour
- 1 teaspoon of almond flour
- 1 teaspoon of psyllium
- 1 teaspoon of baking powder
- 1 egg at room temperature
- 1 teaspoon of extra virgin olive oil or melted butter

NUTRITIONS

Calories: 112 kcal, Gross carbohydrates: 2 g,Protein: 9 g,
Fats: 6 g; Fiber: 5 g, Net carbohydrates: -3 g,
Macro fat: 50 %, Macro proteins: 75 %,
Macro carbohydrates: -25 %

DIRECTIONS

1. Put the dry ingredients in a cup and mix well. In particular, ensure that the baking powder is no longer visible. It helps if you put the baking powder through a (tea) strainer.

2. Now add the egg and the butter. The egg must be at room temperature. If it is not, then place it for about 10 minutes in a bowl with hot tap water.

3. Stir well and let it stand for a while. You will see that there are some bubbles in the batter.

4. Now put the cup in the microwave for 1 minute on the highest setting. When you take the cup out, you want the top of the batter to be dry. If it is still wet, then put it in the microwave for a little longer. (If you put several cups in the microwave at the same time, you may have to extend the time slightly depending on your type of microwave).

5. Once the top is dry, remove the cup from the microwave and turn it on a cutting board. Decide now if you want thick rolls or something thinner. So cut into 2 or 3 or 4 slices. Keep in mind that these slices must fit in your toaster.

6. Now toast the bread slices in your toaster until they are firm but not hard.

7. Your bread is now ready. You can use it immediately or use it for your breakfast or lunch the another day. Spread the butter on it well so that you will get enough fats.

12. Keto Croque Monsieur

PREPARATION

5 MIN

COOKING

7 MIN

SERVES

2

INGREDIENTS

- 2 eggs
- 25 grams of grated cheese
- 25 grams of ham 1 large slice
- 40 ml of cream
- 40 ml of mascarpone
- 30 grams of butter
- Pepper and salt
- Basil leaves, optional, to garnish

NUTRITIONS

Calories: 479 kcal, Gross carbohydrates: 4 g, Protein: 16 g, Fats: 45 g, Net carbohydrates: 4 g, Macro fats: 69 %, Macro proteins: 25 %, Macro carbohydrates: 6 %

DIRECTIONS

1. Carefully crack eggs in a neat bowl, add some salt and pepper.

2. Add the cream, mascarpone and grated cheese and stir together.

3. Melt the butter over a medium heat. The butter must not turn brown. Once the butter has melted, set the heat to low.

4. Add half of the omelette mixture to the frying pan and then immediately place the slice of ham on it. Now pour the rest of the omelette mixture over the ham and then immediately put a lid on it.

5. Allow it to fry for 2-3 minutes over a low heat until the top is slightly firmer.

6. Slide the omelette onto the lid to turn the omelette. Then put the omelette back in the frying pan to fry for another 1-2 minutes on the other side (still on low heat), then put the lid back on the pan.

7. Don't let the omelette cook for too long! It does not matter if it is still liquid. Garnish with a few basil leaves if necessary.

13. Keto Wraps With Cream Cheese And Salmon

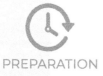

PREPARATION

5 MIN

COOKING

10 MIN

SERVES

2

INGREDIENTS

- 80 grams of cream cheese
- 1 tablespoon of dill or other fresh herbs
- 30 grams of smoked salmon
- 1 egg
- 15 grams of butter
- Pinch of cayenne pepper
- Pepper and salt

NUTRITIONS

Calories: 237, Carbohydrates: 14.7g,
Protein: 15g, Fat: 5g

DIRECTIONS

1. Beat the egg well in a bowl. With 1 egg, you can make two thin wraps in a small frying pan.

2. Melt the butter over a medium heat in a small frying pan. Once the butter has melted, add half of the beaten egg to the pan. Move the pan back and forth so that the entire bottom is covered with a very thin layer of egg. Turn down the heat!

3. Carefully loosen the egg on the edges with a silicone spatula and turn the wafer-thin omelette as soon as the egg is no longer dripping (about 45 seconds to 1 minute). You can do this by sliding it onto a lid or plate and then sliding it back into the pan. Let the other side be cooked for about 30 seconds and then remove from the pan. The omelette must be nice and light yellow. Repeat for the rest of the beaten egg.

4. Once the omelettes are ready, let them cool on a cutting board or plate and make the filling.

5. Cut or cut the dill into small pieces and put in a bowl.

6. Add the cream cheese and the salmon, cut into small pieces. Mix together. Add a tiny bit of cayenne pepper and mix well. Taste immediately and then season with salt and pepper.

7. Spread a layer on the wrap and roll it up. Cut the wrap in half and keep in the fridge until you are ready to eat it.

14. Slow Cooker Chilli

PREPARATION
15 MIN

COOKING
6 HOURS 15 MIN

SERVES
6

INGREDIENTS

- 2 ½ lbs ground beef
- 1 red onion, diced
- 5 cloves garlic, minced
- 1 ½ c celery, diced
- 1 6-ounce can tomato paste
- 1 14.5 oz can diced tomatoes with green chilies
- 1 14.5 oz can stewed tomatoes
- 4 T chili powder
- 2 T ground cumin
- 2 t salt
- 1 t garlic powder
- 1 t onion powder
- 3 t cayenne pepper
- 1 t red pepper flakes

NUTRITIONS

Calories: 137, Carbohydrates: 4.7g,
Protein: 16g, Fat: 5g

DIRECTIONS

1. Cook ground beef in a large skillet.

2. Add onion, garlic, and celery and cook until ground beef browned

3. Drain the fat from the beef

4. Place beef and vegetable mixture into the slow cooker set on a low setting.

5. Add tomatoes and seasonings then stir to mix.

6. Place the lid on the slow cooker and cook on low for 6 hours.

7. Serve with cheese on top if desired. Adjust the red pepper to taste.

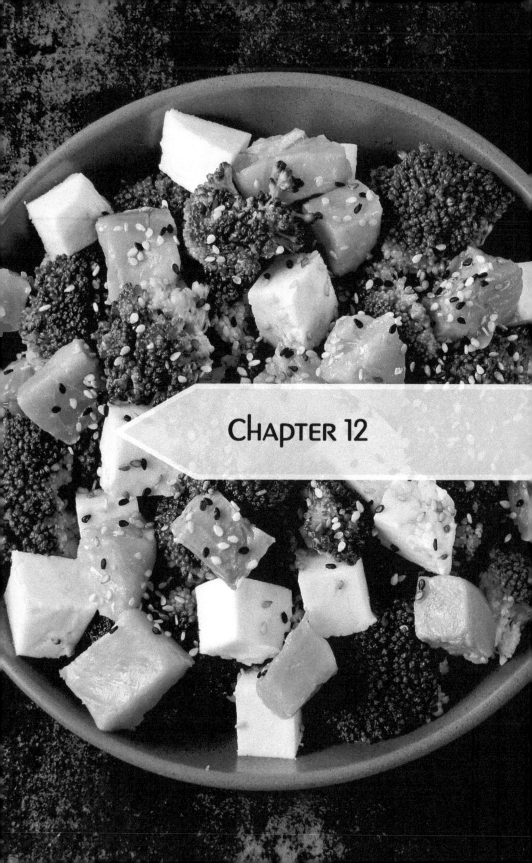

Chapter 12

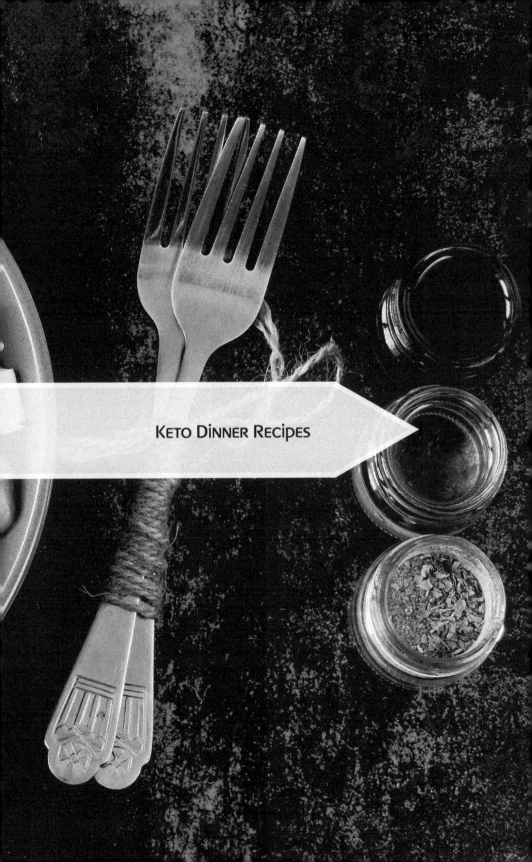

Keto Dinner Recipes

15. Slow Roasting Pork Shoulder

PREPARATION

15 MIN

COOKING

7 HOURS

SERVES

8

INGREDIENTS

- 3 lb. pork shoulder
- 8 garlic cloves, minced
- ½ C. fresh lemon juice
- 2 tbsp. olive oil
- 1 tbsp. low-sodium soy sauce
- 1/3 C. homemade chicken broth

NUTRITIONS

Calories per serving: 537, Carbohydrates: 1.5g, Protein: 40.2g, Fat: 40.1g, Sugar: 0.5g, Sodium: 261mg, Fiber: 0.1g

DIRECTIONS

1. In a nonreactive baking dish, arrange the pork shoulder, fat side up.

2. With the tip of knife, score the fat in a crosshatch pattern.

3. In a bowl, add the garlic, lemon juice, soy sauce and oil and mix well.

4. Place the marinade over pork and coat well.

5. Refrigerate for about 4-6 hours, flipping occasionally.

6. Preheat the oven to 3150 F. Lightly, grease a large roasting pan.

7. With paper towels, wipe marinade off the pork shoulder.

8. Arrange the pork shoulder into prepared roasting pan, fat side up.

9. Roast for about 3 hours.

10. Remove from the oven and pour the broth over the pork shoulder.

11. Roast for about 3-4 hours, basting with pan juices, after every 1 hour.

12. Remove from oven and place the pork shoulder onto a cutting board for about 30 minutes.

13. With a sharp knife, cut the pork shoulder into desired size slices and serve.

16. Garlicky Pork Shoulder

PREPARATION
15 MIN

COOKING
6 HOURS

SERVES
10

INGREDIENTS

- 1 head garlic, peeled and crushed
- ¼ C. fresh rosemary, minced
- 2 tbsp. fresh lemon juice
- 2 tbsp. balsamic vinegar
- 1 (4-lb.) pork shoulder

NUTRITIONS

Calories per serving: 502, Carbohydrates: 2g, Protein: 42.5g,
Fat: 39.1g, Sugar: 0.1g, Sodium: 125mg, Fiber: 0.7g

DIRECTIONS

1. In a bowl, add all the ingredients except pork shoulder and mix well.

2. In a large roasting pan, place the pork shoulder and generously coat with the marinade.

3. With a large plastic wrap, cover the roasting pan and refrigerate to marinate for at least 1-2 hours.

4. Remove the roasting pan from refrigerator.

5. Remove the plastic wrap from roasting pan and keep in room temperature for 1 hour.

6. Preheat the oven to 2750 F.

7. Place the roasting pan into oven and roast for about 6 hours.

8. Remove from the oven and place pork shoulder onto a cutting board for about 30 minutes.

9. With a sharp knife, cut the pork shoulder into desired size slices and serve.

17. Rosemary Pork Roast

PREPARATION
15 MIN

COOKING
60 MIN

SERVES
6

INGREDIENTS

- 1 tbsp. dried rosemary, crushed
- 3 garlic cloves, minced
- Salt and freshly ground black pepper, to taste
- 2 lb. boneless pork loin roast
- ¼ C. olive oil
- 1/3 C. homemade chicken broth

NUTRITIONS

Calories per serving: 294, Carbohydrates: 0.9g,
Protein: 40g, Fat: 13.9g, Sugar: 0.1g,
Sodium: 156mg, Fiber: 0.3g

DIRECTIONS

1. Preheat the oven to 3500 F. Lightly, grease a roasting pan.

2. In a small bowl, add rosemary, garlic, salt and black pepper and with the back of spoon, crush the mixture to form a paste.

3. With a sharp knife, pierce the pork loin at many places.

4. Press the half of rosemary mixture into the cuts.

5. Add oil in the bowl with remaining rosemary mixture and stir to combine.

6. Rub the pork with rosemary mixture generously.

7. Arrange the pork loin into the prepared roasting pan.

8. Roast for about 1 hour, flipping and coating with the pan juices occasionally.

9. Remove the roasting pan from oven. Transfer the pork into a serving platter.

10. Place the roasting pan over medium heat.

11. Add the broth and cook for about 3-5 minutes, stirring to lose the brown bits from pan.

12. Pour sauce over pork and serve.

18. Winter Season Pork Dish

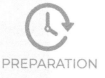
PREPARATION
15 MIN

COOKING
120 MIN

SERVES
8

INGREDIENTS

- 24 oz. sauerkraut
- 2 lb. pork roast
- Salt and freshly ground black pepper, to taste
- ¼ C. unsalted butter
- ½ yellow onion, sliced thinly
- 14 oz. precooked kielbasa, sliced into ½-inch rounds

NUTRITIONS

Calories per serving: 417, Carbohydrates: 6.3g,
Protein: 39g, Fat: 25g, Sugar: 2g,
Sodium: 1200mg, Fiber: 3g

DIRECTIONS

1. Preheat the oven to 3250 F.

2. Drain the sauerkraut, reserving about 1 C. of liquid.

3. Lightly, season the pork roast with salt and black pepper.

4. In a heavy-bottomed skillet, melt the butter over high heat and sear the pork for about 5-6 minutes per side.

5. With a slotted spoon, transfer the pork onto a plate.

6. In the bottom of a casserole, place half of sauerkraut and onion slices.

7. Place the seared pork roast and kielbasa pieces on top.

8. Top with the remaining sauerkraut and onion slices.

9. Pour the reserved sauerkraut liquid into casserole dish.

10. Cover the casserole dish tightly and bake for about 2 hours.

11. Remove from the oven and with tongs, transfer the pork roast onto a cutting board for at least 15 minutes.

12. With a sharp knife, cut the pork roast into desired size slices.

13. Divide the pork slices onto serving plates and serve alongside the sauerkraut mixture.

19. Celebrating Pork Tenderloin

PREPARATION

15 MIN

COOKING

40 MIN

SERVES

6

INGREDIENTS

- For Pork Tenderloin:
- 3 medium garlic cloves, minced
- 3 tsp. dried rosemary, crushed
- ½ tsp. cayenne pepper
- Salt and freshly ground black pepper, to taste
- 2 lb. pork tenderloin
- For Blueberry Sauce:
- 1 tbsp. olive oil
- 1 medium yellow onion, chopped
- ½ tsp. Erythritol
- 1/3 C. organic apple cider vinegar
- 1½ C. fresh blueberries
- ½ tsp. dried thyme, crushed
- Salt and freshly ground black pepper, to taste

NUTRITIONS

Calories per serving: 276, Carbohydrates: 9g;
Protein: 40g, Fat: 8g, Sugar: 5g,
Sodium: 116mg, Fiber: 2g

DIRECTIONS

1. Preheat the oven to 4000 F. Grease a roasting pan.

2. For pork: in a bowl, mix together all the ingredients except pork.

3. Rub the pork with garlic mixture evenly.

4. Place the pork into prepared roasting pan.

5. Roast for about 25 minutes or until desired doneness.

6. Meanwhile, for sauce; in a pan, heat the oil over medium-high heat and sauté the onion for about 4-5 minutes.

7. Stir in the remaining ingredients and cook for about 7-8 minutes or until desired thickness, stirring frequently.

8. Remove the roasting pan from oven and place the pork tenderloin onto a cutting board for about 10-15 minutes.

9. With a sharp knife, cut the pork tenderloin into desired size slices and serve with the topping of blueberry sauce.

20. Mustard Pork Tenderloin

PREPARATION
15 MIN

COOKING
30 MIN

SERVES
4

INGREDIENTS

- 1 tsp. fresh rosemary, minced
- 1 garlic clove, minced
- 1 tbsp. fresh lemon juice
- 1 tbsp. olive oil
- 1 tsp. Dijon mustard
- 1 tsp. powdered Swerve
- Salt and freshly ground black pepper, to taste
- 1 lb. pork tenderloin
- ¼ C. blue cheese, crumbled

Calories per serving: 227, Carbohydrates: 2g,
Protein: 37g, Fat: 10g, Sugar: 0.5g,
Sodium: 236mg, Fiber: 0.1g

DIRECTIONS

1. Preheat oven to 4000 F. Grease a large rimmed baking sheet.

2. In a large bowl, add all the ingredients except the pork tenderloin and cheese and beat until well combined.

3. Add the pork tenderloin and coat with the mixture generously.

4. Arrange the pork tenderloin onto the prepared baking sheet.

5. Bake for about 20-22 minutes.

6. Remove from the oven and place the pork tenderloin onto a cutting board for about 5 minutes.

7. With a sharp knife, cut the pork tenderloin into ¾-inch thick slices and serve with the topping of cheese.

21. Succulent Pork Tenderloin

PREPARATION
20 MIN

COOKING
60 MIN

SERVES
4

INGREDIENTS

- 1 lb. pork tenderloin
- 1 tbsp. unsalted butter
- 2 tsp. garlic, minced
- 2 oz. fresh spinach
- 4 oz. cream cheese, softened
- 1 tsp. liquid smoke
- Salt and freshly ground black pepper, to taste

NUTRITIONS

Calories per serving: 315, Carbohydrates: 3g,
Protein: 43g, Fat: 23g, Sugar: 0.5g,
Sodium: 261mg, Fiber: 0.1g

DIRECTIONS

1. Preheat the oven to 3500 F. Line casserole dish with a piece of the foil.

2. Arrange the pork tenderloin between 2 plastic wraps and with a meat tenderizer, pound until flat.

3. Carefully, cut the edges of tenderloin to shape into a rectangle.

4. In a large skillet, melt the butter over medium heat and sauté the garlic for about 1 minute.

5. Add the spinach, cream cheese, liquid smoke, salt and black pepper and cook for about 3-4 minutes.

6. Remove from the heat and set aside to cool slightly.

7. Place the spinach mixture onto pork tenderloin about ½-inch from the edges.

8. Carefully roll tenderloin into a log and secure with toothpicks.

9. Arrange the tenderloin into the prepared casserole dish, seam-side down.

10. Bake for about 1¼ hours.

11. Remove from the oven and let it cool slightly before cutting.

12. Cut the tenderloin into desired sized slices and serve.

22. Simple Ever Rib Roast

PREPARATION
15 MIN

COOKING
60 MIN

SERVES
15

INGREDIENTS

- 10 garlic cloves, minced
- 2 tsp. dried thyme, crushed
- 2 tbsp. olive oil
- Salt and freshly ground black pepper, to taste
- 1 (10-lb.) grass-fed prime rib roast

NUTRITIONS

Calories per serving: 500, Carbohydrates: 1g,
Protein: 60g, Fat: 26g, Sugar: 0.5g,
Sodium: 200mg, Fiber: 0.1g

DIRECTIONS

1. In a bowl, mix together all the ingredients except rib roast.

2. In a large roasting pan, place the rib roast, fatty side up.

3. Coat the rib roast with garlic mixture evenly.

4. Set aside to marinate at the room temperature for at least 1 hour.

5. Preheat the oven to 5000 F.

6. Roast for about 20 minutes.

7. Now, reduce the temperature of oven to 3250 F.

8. Roast for 65-75 minutes.

9. Remove from oven and place the roast onto a cutting board for about 10-15 minutes before slicing.

10. With a sharp knife cut the rib roast in desired sized slices and serve.

23. Family Dinner Tenderloin

PREPARATION
15 MIN

COOKING
30 MIN

SERVES
6

INGREDIENTS

- 4 garlic cloves, minced
- ½ C. fresh parsley, chopped
- 1/3 C. fresh oregano, chopped
- 2 tbsp. fresh thyme, chopped
- 2 tbsp. fresh rosemary, chopped
- 2 tsp. fresh lemon zest, grated
- 6 tbsp. olive oil
- 2 tbsp. fresh lemon juice
- ½ tsp. red pepper flakes
- Salt and freshly ground black pepper, to taste
- 1¾ lb. grass-fed beef tenderloin, silver skin removed

NUTRITIONS

Calories per serving: 420, Carbohydrates: 5.2g,
Protein: 40g, Fat: 27g, Sugar: 0.5g,
Sodium: 121mg, Fiber: 3g

DIRECTIONS

1. In a large bowl, add all the ingredients except the beef tenderloin and mix well.

2. Add the beef tenderloin and coat with the herb mixture generously.

3. Refrigerate to marinate for about 30-45 minutes.

4. Preheat the oven to 4250 F.

5. Remove the beef tenderloin from the bowl and arrange onto a baking sheet.

6. Bake for about 30 minutes.

7. Remove from the oven and place the beef tenderloin onto a cutting board for about 15-20 minutes before slicing.

8. With a sharp knife, cut the beef tenderloin into desired sized slices and serve.

Chapter 13

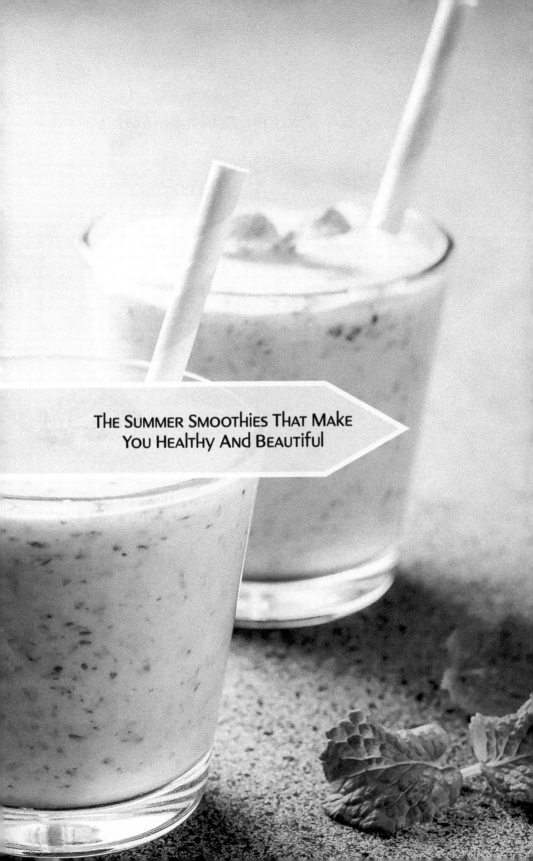

The Summer Smoothies That Make
You Healthy And Beautiful

24. Coconut Green Smoothie

PREPARATION
15 MIN

COOKING
30 MIN

SERVES
6

This smoothie has coconut oil and coconut milk as a wonderful pick-me-up when you need a shot of fiber. Enjoy the fresh coconut flavor that is balanced with matcha. It is a refreshing drink for any time.

INGREDIENTS

- ⅔ c slightly defrosted frozen chopped spinach
- ½ avocado
- 1 T coconut oil
- ½ t matcha powder
- 1 T monk fruit sweetener
- ½ c coconut milk (from the dairy section, not canned)
- ⅔ c water
- ½ cup of ice

Calories per serving: 315, Carbohydrates: 3g,
Protein: 43g, Fat: 23g, Sugar: 0.5g,
Sodium: 261mg, Fiber: 0.1g

DIRECTIONS

1. Add all ingredients except the ice into a blender. Blend until everything is blended well.

2. Pulse in the ice until it is evenly distributed.

3. Pour into a glass.

This smoothie is good for fiber and fat. You can add flaxseed or softened chia seeds to the smoothie for additional fiber and nutrients. Fresh spinach can be used and may be substituted with fresh or frozen kale.

25. Strawberry Smoothie

PREPARATION
15 MIN

COOKING
30 MIN

SERVES
6

Add a touch of sweetness to your day with this strawberry smoothie. This smoothie is good enough for dessert. If you want to add some fiber and protein, try adding chia seeds that have been softened in water. 2 tablespoons of chia will add 139 calories, 1 gram of carbohydrate, 4 grams of protein, and 9 grams of fat.

INGREDIENTS

- ¼ c heavy cream
- ¾ c unsweetened vanilla almond milk
- 2 t stevia
- ½ c frozen strawberries (whole or sliced)
- ½ c ice (preferably crushed)

NUTRITIONS

Calories per serving: 352, Carbohydrates: 2g;
Protein: 42.5g, Fat: 42g, Sugar: 0.1g,
Sodium: 152mg, Fiber: 0.7g

DIRECTIONS

1.   Blend ingredients in a blender until blended well.

2.   Pour into a tall glass.

3.   Serve.

26. Keto Mojito

PREPARATION
15 MIN

COOKING
30 MIN

SERVES
6

Yes! There are keto-friendly cocktails. It takes a little preparation; stevia is used instead of sugar, but you don't need a blender. Muddling the mint leaves releases the mint fragrance and provides the minty backdrop for this refreshing drink. This is an easy recipe that is festive and interactive (muddling) for a fun part beverage.

INGREDIENTS

- 4 fresh mint leaves
- 2 T fresh lime Juice
- 2 t stevia
- Ice
- 1.5 oz shot of white rum
- splash club soda or plain seltzer
- fresh mint as garnish

Calories: 109, Carbohydrates: 2g

DIRECTIONS

1. Muddle the mint, lime juice, and stevia for 10 seconds in the glass in which the drink will be served.

2. Fill the glass with ice, either cubed or crushed.

3. Pour the shot of vodka over the ice.

4. Add club soda to fill the glass

5. Garnish with a mint leaf.

You may want to strain the drink after muddling to remove the broken mint leaves, so they don't get in the way of enjoying the drink. You can substitute vodka or gin for rum.

27. Chocolate Coconut Keto Smoothie Bowl

PREPARATION
15 MIN

COOKING
30 MIN

SERVES
6

INGREDIENTS

- 1/3 cup vanilla protein powder
- 1 tbsp cocoa powder
- 1/4 cup walnuts
- 1/4 cup walnuts
- 1/2 cup almond milk
- 1 tbsp coconut oil
- 3 cup crushed ice
- Sweetener

NUTRITIONS

Calories per serving: 352, Carbohydrates: 2g,
Protein: 42.5g, Fat: 42g, Sugar: 0.1g
Sodium: 152mg, Fiber: 0.7g

DIRECTIONS

1. Take a blender pour almond milk, protein powder, cocoa powder, sweetener and ice, blend the ingredients well.

2. Now add coconut oil xanthan gum and blend until it increases in volume.

3. Pour it into bowl adds fruits and nuts and serves.

Conclusion

For some people, the ketogenic get-healthy plan is a phenomenal path for weight reduction. It is extraordinary and permits the person on the eating routine to devour an eating plan, which incorporates nourishments that you probably won't anticipate.

Along these lines, the ketogenic diet, or keto, is an eating plan that comprises of high fat and low carbs. Exactly what number of diet programs are there in which you can set up the free day with eggs and bacon, huge amounts of it, at that point take chicken wings for lunch and broccoli and steak for dinner.

That could sound too extraordinary to be in any way precise for some. Adequately on this specific eating routine, this is a phenomenal day of eating and you followed the rules totally with that supper program.

At whatever point you expend a little amount of sugars, the body is put into a condition of ketosis. This means the body can consume fat for vitality. Exactly how little of various carbs would you need to devour that can go into ketosis?Effectively, it differs for every person, though it is a safe option to remain under twenty-five total carbs. Most suggest that when you are in the "induction phase" that happens when you are really putting the body into ketosis, you must remain under ten total carbs.

Something to stress about when going on the ketogenic diet plan is a thing known as "keto flu. You will feel fatigued and you might have a headache. It will not last lengthy. If you are feeling by doing this, make certain you receive a lot of rest and water to overcome it.

Intermittent fasting has transformed into a most loved strategy to utilize your body's normal fat-copying ability to get in shape in a quick time. All things considered, numerous people wish to know, accomplishes discontinuous fasting work and exactly how precisely will it work?

At whatever point you go for a drawn out timeframe with no eating, the body changes the manner by which it produces proteins and hormones, which could be useful for weight reduction. These are the essential fasting benefits and the manner in which they achieve those advantages.

Hormones structure the establishment of metabolic stacks like the speed at which you consume off muscle versus fat. Development hormone is made by the body and energizes the breakdown of fat inside the body to give vitality.If you fast for quite a while, the body starts to improve the development hormone creation. Also, fasting attempts to diminish the amount of insulin contained in the circulatory system, ensuring that the body consumes fat as opposed to putting away it.

A momentary quick which keeps going 12-72 hours expands the metabolic procedure and adrenaline levels, making you support the quantity of calories consumed. Moreover, the individuals who quick furthermore acknowledge higher vitality through improved adrenaline, pushing them to not look depleted in spite of the fact that they are not getting calories regularly. While you may feel as fasting must prompt diminished vitality, the whole body makes up for this particular, guaranteeing a more unhealthy consuming daily schedule.

Almost all people that eat each 3-5 hours chiefly consume sugar as opposed to fat. Fasting for a significant stretch moves the digestion to losing fat. By the decision of a 24-hour fasting day, the body has just spent glycogen traders in two or three hours and has now invested around eighteen of the energy consuming by additional fat stores inside the body.

For anyone who is continually profitable, be that as it may, battles with weight reduction, irregular fasting can make it conceivable to support weight reduction without being compelled to increase an exercise design or definitely modify an eating routine program.An additional advantage of intermittent fasting is the fact that it resets an individual's body. Getting one day or even so without consuming changes an individual's craving, causing them to not really feel as starved after a while.

When you wrestle with consistently desiring food, intermittent fasting can assist your body to adjust to periods of refusing to eat and enable you to not really feel hungry continuously. Many people notice they begin eating healthier plus more controlled diets whenever they fast intermittently 1 day a week.

Intermittent fasting differs but is frequently recommended for approximately 1 day each week. During this working day, a person could have a nutrient-filled smoothie or any other low-calorie drink. As the entire body changes to an intermittent fasting program, this generally is not essential.

Intermittent fasting helps you to lessen body fat stores effortlessly in the entire body, by changing over the metabolism for breaking down body fat rather than muscle or sugar.

It has been used by many people effectively and it is a simple way to make an advantageous change. For anybody that struggles with stubborn fat and it is tired of regular dieting, intermittent fasting provides an effective and easy choice for weight loss and a healthier way of life.

If these two dieting patterns sound like the diet types, you will be interested in, then WHAT ARE YOU WAITING FOR?